Headache Disorders: New Advances in Management and Treatment Strategies

Headache Disorders: New Advances in Management and Treatment Strategies

Guest Editors

Andreas A. Argyriou
Vikelis Michail
Emmanouil V. Dermitzakis

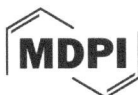

Basel • Beijing • Wuhan • Barcelona • Belgrade • Novi Sad • Cluj • Manchester

Guest Editors

Andreas A. Argyriou
Neurology Department
Agios Andreas State General
Hospital of Patras
Patras
Greece

Vikelis Michail
Headache Clinic
Mediterraneo Hospital
Glyfada
Greece

Emmanouil V. Dermitzakis
Euromedica General Clinic
Thessaloniki
Greece

Editorial Office
MDPI AG
Grosspeteranlage 5
4052 Basel, Switzerland

This is a reprint of the Special Issue, published open access by the journal *Journal of Clinical Medicine* (ISSN 2077-0383), freely accessible at: https://www.mdpi.com/journal/jcm/special_issues/90L7N0D357.

For citation purposes, cite each article independently as indicated on the article page online and as indicated below:

Lastname, A.A.; Lastname, B.B. Article Title. *Journal Name* **Year**, *Volume Number*, Page Range.

ISBN 978-3-7258-4347-3 (Hbk)
ISBN 978-3-7258-4348-0 (PDF)
https://doi.org/10.3390/books978-3-7258-4348-0

© 2025 by the authors. Articles in this book are Open Access and distributed under the Creative Commons Attribution (CC BY) license. The book as a whole is distributed by MDPI under the terms and conditions of the Creative Commons Attribution-NonCommercial-NoDerivs (CC BY-NC-ND) license (https://creativecommons.org/licenses/by-nc-nd/4.0/).

Contents

Andreas A. Argyriou, Emmanouil V. Dermitzakis, Georgia Xiromerisiou, Dimitrios Rallis, Panagiotis Soldatos, Pantelis Litsardopoulos and Michail Vikelis
Predictors of Response to Fremanezumab in Migraine Patients with at Least Three Previous Preventive Failures: Post Hoc Analysis of a Prospective, Multicenter, Real-World Greek Registry
Reprinted from: *Journal of Clinical Medicine* **2023**, *12*, 3218, https://doi.org/10.3390/jcm12093218   1

Michail Vikelis, Emmanouil V. Dermitzakis, Georgia Xiromerisiou, Dimitrios Rallis, Panagiotis Soldatos, Pantelis Litsardopoulos, et al.
Effects of Fremanezumab on Psychiatric Comorbidities in Difficult-to-Treat Patients with Chronic Migraine: Post Hoc Analysis of a Prospective, Multicenter, Real-World Greek Registry
Reprinted from: *Journal of Clinical Medicine* **2023**, *12*, 4526, https://doi.org/10.3390/jcm12134526   11

Thomas Berk, Stephen Silberstein and Peter McAllister
A Novel Virtual-Based Comprehensive Clinical Approach to Headache Care
Reprinted from: *Journal of Clinical Medicine* **2023**, *12*, 5349, https://doi.org/10.3390/jcm12165349   21

Nader G. Zalaquett, Elio Salameh, Jonathan M. Kim, Elham Ghanbarian, Karen Tawk and Mehdi Abouzari
The Dawn and Advancement of the Knowledge of the Genetics of Migraine
Reprinted from: *Journal of Clinical Medicine* **2024**, *13*, 2701, https://doi.org/10.3390/jcm13092701   29

Anat Horev, Sapir Aharoni-Bar, Mark Katson, Erez Tsumi, Tamir Regev, Yair Zlotnik, et al.
Predictors of Headaches and Quality of Life in Women with Ophthalmologically Resolved Idiopathic Intracranial Hypertension
Reprinted from: *Journal of Clinical Medicine* **2024**, *13*, 3971, https://doi.org/10.3390/jcm13133971   59

Marina Stoupa Hadidi, Murad Rasheed, Yanal M. Bisharat, Heba H. Al Helou, Hussam A. El Aina, Hala M. Batayneh, et al.
Efficacy of Desvenlafaxine in Reducing Migraine Frequency and Severity: A Retrospective Study
Reprinted from: *Journal of Clinical Medicine* **2024**, *13*, 5156, https://doi.org/10.3390/jcm13175156   71

Abdulrahim Saleh Alrasheed, Taif Mansour Almaqboul, Reem Ali Alshamrani, Noor Mohammad AlMohish and Majed Mohammad Alabdali
Safety and Efficacy of Atogepant for the Preventive Treatment of Migraines in Adults: A Systematic Review and Meta-Analysis
Reprinted from: *Journal of Clinical Medicine* **2024**, *13*, 6713, https://doi.org/10.3390/jcm13226713   82

Ignazio Leale, Vincenzo Di Stefano, Angelo Torrente, Paolo Alonge, Roberto Monastero, Michele Roccella, et al.
Telecoaching and Migraine: Digital Approach to Physical Activity in Migraine Management. A Scoping Review
Reprinted from: *Journal of Clinical Medicine* **2025**, *14*, 861, https://doi.org/10.3390/jcm14030861   101

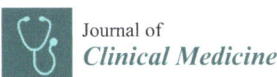

Article

Predictors of Response to Fremanezumab in Migraine Patients with at Least Three Previous Preventive Failures: Post Hoc Analysis of a Prospective, Multicenter, Real-World Greek Registry

Andreas A. Argyriou [1,*], Emmanouil V. Dermitzakis [2], Georgia Xiromerisiou [3], Dimitrios Rallis [4], Panagiotis Soldatos [5], Pantelis Litsardopoulos [1] and Michail Vikelis [6]

1. Headache Outpatient Clinic, Neurology Department, Agios Andreas State General Hospital of Patras, 26335 Patras, Greece; pantelis84@hotmail.com
2. Euromedica General Clinic, 54645 Thessaloniki, Greece; manolis.dermitzakis@gmail.com
3. Department of Neurology, School of Medicine, University of Thessaly, 41221 Larissa, Greece; georgiaxiromerisiou@gmail.com
4. Department of Neurology, Tzaneio General Hospital of Piraeus, 18536 Athens, Greece; jimrallis@hotmail.com
5. Private Practice, 24100 Kalamata, Greece; soldatosp@gmail.com
6. Headache Clinic, Mediterraneo Hospital, 16673 Glyfada, Greece; mvikelis@headaches.gr
* Correspondence: andargyriou@yahoo.gr

Abstract: Objective: To define, in a real-world population of patients with high-frequency episodic (HFEM) or chronic migraine (CM), the predictive role of socio-demographic or phenotypic profiling of responders to fremanezumab. Patients and methods: Two-hundred and four adult fremanezumab-treated patients with either HFEM or CM, who failed to at least three preventive treatments, provided data at baseline on several individual socio-demographic and phenotypic variables. These variables were analyzed for their ability to independently predict the response (50–74% response rates) or super-response ($\geq$ 75% response rates) to fremanezumab. Patients were followed from 3–18 months of fremanezumab exposure. Results: The main finding to emerge from univariate analyses was that three baseline socio-demographic/clinical variables, i.e., age group 41–70 years ($p = 0.02$); female gender ($p = 0.03$); patients with HFEM ($p = 0.001$), and three clinical phenotypic variables, i.e., strict unilateral pain ($p = 0.05$); pain in the ophthalmic trigeminal branch ($p = 0.04$); and the "imploding" quality of pain ($p = 0.05$), were significantly related to fremanezumab response. However, in multivariate analysis, only HFEM ($p = 0.02$), the presence of strict unilateral ($p = 0.03$), and pain location in the ophthalmic trigeminal branch ($p = 0.036$) were independently associated with good fremanezumab response. Allodynia ($p = 0.04$) was the only clinical predictive variable of super-responsiveness to fremanezumab. Conclusions: A precise phenotypic profiling with identification of pain characteristics consistent with peripheral and/or central sensitization might reliably predict the responsiveness to fremanezumab in migraine prophylaxis.

Keywords: CGRP; monoclonal antibodies; fremanezumab; phenotypes; predictors; response; episodic migraine; chronic migraine

1. Introduction

The introduction of monoclonal antibodies (MAbs), specifically targeting the calcitonin gene-related peptide (CGRP) or its receptor (anti-CGRP MAbs), has revolutionized the prophylactic treatment of migraine [1]. Their mode of action is based on the ability to selectively inhibit the activation of the trigeminovascular pain pathway [2,3].

Fremanezumab, a humanized anti-CGRP Mab with abilities to selectively target the CGRP ligand and to prevent its binding to the receptor in the trigeminal ganglion and meningeal nociceptors [4], has demonstrated a favorable benefit-risk ratio in large regulatory placebo-controlled randomized clinical trials [5] and was approved in 2018–2019 by international drug agencies for the prophylactic treatment of both episodic (EM) and chronic migraine (CM). After the release of formal approval, several real-world studies worldwide validated its excellent safety/tolerability profile [6,7], marking the onset of a new era in migraine prophylaxis, compared to the usual standard of care with the use of orally taken beta blockers, antiepileptics and tricyclics [8].

Fremanezumab has been commercially available in Greece for migraine prophylaxis since 2020, while reimbursement came in 2021 for patients with high frequency EM (HFEM: 8–14 days/month) or CM, having previously failed to at least three preventives, including OnabotulinumtoxinA (only in CM patients). We have recently reported the outcome of the first prospective real-world study from Greece on the efficacy/safety of fremanezumab in difficult-to-treat migraine patients, and demonstrated that it was able to reduce, by at least 50%, the monthly headache days (MHD) in about two-third of the 204 enrolled patients with either HFEM or CM. As a result of this beneficial effect, patients had less disability and improved quality of life [9].

Our results are generally in agreement with previous evidence showing that up to one-third of patients remain unresponsive to preventative therapies with anti-CGRP MAbs, including fremanezumab [10]. Towards the latter evidence, and also considering the lack of a reliable disease biomarker, it is important to identify clinical predictors of response to anti-CGRP MAbs in order to guide tailored and personalized therapeutic protocols for each patient so as to optimize good clinical outcomes as well as resources allocation [11].

Although there is evidence to suggest that some baseline demographic and clinical characteristics, as well as phenotypic features, might be able to predict the responsiveness to anti-CGRP MAbs, the issue still remains only partly elucidated because of mixed results and common heterogeneities in findings reported from available studies [12–15]. Another important aspect that needs to be further addressed is to define the profile of patients who experience super-response to anti-CGRP MAbs, especially if potential predictors to these outcomes are to be identified for these individuals.

Therefore, the aim of this post hoc analysis of data extracted from a prospective, multicenter, Greek registry is to define, in a real-world population of patients with HFEM or CM, the predictive role of socio-demographic and phenotypic profiling of responders ($\geq$ 50% MHD reduction) or super-responders ($\geq$ 75% MHD reduction) to fremanezumab.

2. Materials and Methods

Two-hundred and four adult patients with a definite diagnosis of either HFEM or CM [16], who received treatment with at least 3 monthly cycles or 1 per trimester cycle of fremanezumab at six different Greek hospitals or headache-focused private clinics, took part in this post hoc analysis. The study protocol was approved by the Institutional Review Board of "Agios Andreas" Patras General Hospital, and an informed consent was obtained from each patient before being included into the study, in accordance with the requirements of the Declaration of Helsinki.

Eligibility was confirmed by a protocol-specific checklist, while the inclusion and exclusion criteria have been previously described in detail [9]. Briefly, patients had to suffer from either HFEM or CM with or without aura or medication overuse headache (MOH) and be scheduled to receive prophylactic treatment with fremanezumab, as per the approved indication/contraindication [17] and current standard Greek clinical practice and national reimbursement policies. Anti-CGRP MAbs naïve patients received subcutaneous fremanezumab (Ajovy® 225 mg/pf-syr, Teva Pharma-Hellas) 225 mg monthly (every 28–30 days) or 675 mg quarterly (every 90 days) for at least 3 months (12 weeks) before establishing the response rates. Hence, patients were followed from 3–18 months of fremanezumab exposure.

The following socio-demographic, clinical variables, and phenotypic characteristics were carefully collected at baseline and were then analyzed for their ability to predict the response to fremanezumab, in line with previous relevant publications [14,18]: gender;

age groups in years (41–70 vs. 18–40); migraine type (HFEM vs. CM); BMI status (normal [<24.9] vs. overweight/obese [>25]); number of failed preventives (3–5 vs. 6–7); duration of migraine diagnosis (2–15 vs. above 15 years), presence (yes/no) of MOH; aura; family history and comorbidities, the latter either psychiatric or gastrointestinal. Additionally, patients were asked to report the presence of strict unilateral pain (pain never felt on the other side of the head) vs. alternating side; allodynia, i.e., pain resulting from application of a non-noxious stimulus (yes/no); pain in ophthalmic trigeminal branch (yes/no); prodromal dopaminergic symptoms, i.e., mood changes, yawning, somnolence, drowsiness, food craving (yes/no); unilateral autonomic symptoms, i.e., eye redness, lacrimation, nasal congestion, rhinorrhea, eyelid edema, facial edema, forehead and facial sweating, miosis, ptosis (yes/no); quality of pain (imploding vs. exploding pain); response to triptans, defined as headache resolution within 2 h after triptan intake (yes/no); presence of known migraine triggers, including stress, irregular sleep schedule, specific food/alcohol/caffeine consumption, weather changes, dehydration, and luminous and olfactory stimuli (yes/no); and pericranial muscle tenderness (yes/no).

After the first fremanezumab administration, patients completed a daily headache diary (compliance was set to at least 80% of total monthly days) in paper format, and based on the corresponding recordings, compared to those obtained pre-treatment, we divided them in three groups: non-responders (<50% reduction in MHD); responders (50–74% reduction in MHD) and super-responders ($\geq$75% reduction in MHD). Migraine patients were defined as responders or super-responders if they experience either a >50% or a >75% decrease, respectively, in MHD or in the monthly number of moderate/severe headache days during the last 4 weeks of treatment, compared to baseline. Patients who had a decrease in MHD ranging from 26 to 49%, compared to baseline, are defined as non-responders, while a full non-responder is a patient who experiences a <25% decrease in MHD [19]. For the purpose of our study the latter two groups (non-responders and full non-responders) were merged into one group as "non-responders".

We then compared the above-mentioned baseline socio-demographic and clinical characteristics, as well as phenotypic profiling, between non-responders vs. responders and responders vs. super-responders in order to define the predictors of response at $\geq$50% and at $\geq$75% to fremanezumab.

Statistical Analysis

To identify predictors of response to fremanezumab, we performed a univariate analysis using baseline demographic and clinical characteristics of their migraine. Patients who responded to fremanezumab, defined as an at least 50% reduction in their MHD, and non-responders (<50% MHD reduction) were compared using the two-sided chi square test with Yate's correction. The same statistical test was performed to compare patients with response (50–74% MHD reduction) vs. super-response ($\geq$75% MHD reduction) to fremanezumab. To assess independency, all significant variables in univariate analysis were then entered into a backward multivariate logistic regression analysis. All tests were two-tailed and statistical significance was set at the $p < 0.05$ level. Statistical analysis was performed using SPSS for Windows (release 27.0; SPSS Inc., Chicago, IL, USA).

3. Results

The flow chart, as well as the demographic and baseline clinical migraine characteristics of our study sample included in this post hoc analysis, are described in detail in our primary publication that contained our results on the efficacy/safety of fremanezumab in migraine prophylaxis [9]. Briefly, there were 210 patients initially enrolled, with the majority of them to be able to complete the study. There were 6 cases of early withdrawal from the study for reasons including, lost to follow-up (n = 3); cases remained in significant remission and individually decided not to continue treatment (n = 2), as well as one case of pregnancy. As such, of a total of 204 fremanezumab-treated patients for either HFEM (n = 97; 47.5%) or CM (n = 107; 52.4%), after having previously failed a median of

5 preventives, 171 (83.8%) were females, and they had a median age of 47.5 years. The majority (n = 131; 64.3%) of them had a normal BMI of <24.9 and were diagnosed with concurrent MOH (n = 122; 59.8%). Psychiatric comorbidities were also common (n = 121; 59.3%). A total of 148 patients (81/97; 83.5% with HFEM and 67/107; 62.6% CM patients) obtained an at least 50% reduction in MHD, compared to baseline, and were counted as treatment responders.

3.1. Comparison of Baseline Demographic and Clinical Characteristics as Well as Phenotypic Profiling between Responders vs. Non-Responders to Fremanezumab

Concerning the comparison in baseline demographics and clinical features, the responders were more frequently females (p = 0.03), aged between 41–70 years (p = 0.02), who received fremanezumab for HFEM (p = 0.001) than non-responders. The rest of the baseline demographic and clinical data were well balanced between the two groups, as none of the analyzed variables were found to have a statistically significant association with occurrence of response vs. non-response to fremanezumab, including the family history of migraine; BMI status; the number of previously failed preventives; the duration of migraine diagnosis; and the occurrence of MOH, aura, or other major comorbidities (Table 1).

Table 1. Demographic and baseline disease's clinical data in responders (at least 50% reduction in MHD) vs. non-responders (<50% MHD reduction) to fremanezumab. p values in bold indicates statistical significance.

Predictors	Responders n = 148		Non-Responders n = 56		O.R (95% CI)	p Value
	N	%	N	%		
Age in years 41–70 vs. 18–40	95	64.2	21	37.5	1.2 (0.8–1.6)	**0.02**
Gender Females vs. Males	131	88.5	40	71.4	3.2 (1.1–9.5)	**0.03**
Migraine type HFEM vs. CM	81	54.7	16	28.6	7.3 (3.1–8.6)	**0.001**
BMI status						
Normal (<24.9) vs. Overweight/obese (>25)	98	66.2	33	58.9	0.7 (0.4–1.4)	0.332
Failed preventives (n) 3–5 vs. 6–7	65	43.9	20	35.7	0.8 (0.3–1.5)	0.473
Duration in migraine diagnosis (years) 2–15 vs. above 15	74	50	21	37.5	0.9 (0.7–1.2)	0.374
MOH Yes vs. No	90	60.8	32	57.1	0.6 (0.2–1.9)	0.432
Aura Yes vs. No	19	12.8	10	17.8	0.6 (0.3–1.2)	0.3
Family History Yes vs. No	63	42.5	31	53.5	0.8 (0.7–1.1)	0.12
Comorbidities Yes vs. No						
Psychiatric	85	57.4	38	67.8	0.6 (0.3–1.2)	0.151
Gastrointestinal	28	18.9	13	23.2	0.9 (0.8–1.1)	0.513

After univariate analysis, three variables extracted from the phenotypic clinical profile of patients were related to higher rates of response to fremanezumab and thus to favorable outcomes. The responders presented more frequent strict unilateral pain (odds ratio [OR]: 1.8; 95% confidence interval [CI]: 1.2–3.9; $p = 0.05$) or pain in the ophthalmic trigeminal branch (OR: 3.6; 95% confidence interval [CI]: 1.9–7.1; $p = 0.04$), while the quality of their pain was more frequently described as being "imploding" (OR: 1.7; 95% CI: 0.9–3.1; $p = 0.05$), compared to non-responders (Table 2).

Table 2. Incidence of various clinical predictors in migraine patients with response (at least 50% reduction in MHD) vs. non-response (<50% MHD reduction) to fremanezumab.

Predictors	Responders n = 148		Non-Responders n = 56		O.R (95% CI)	p Value
	N	%	N	%		
Strict unilateral pain	60	40.5	15	26.8	1.8 (1.2–3.9)	**0.05**
Allodynia	52	35.1	13	23.2	1.5 (0.6–3.3)	0.071
Pain in ophthalmic trigeminal branch	30	20.3	5	8.9	3.6 (1.9–7.1)	**0.04**
Prodromal Dopaminergic symptoms	85	57.4	25	44.6	0.6 (0.4–1.2)	0.361
Unilateral Autonomic symptoms	56	37.8	15	26.8	0.8 (0.7–1.5)	0.117
Imploding vs. exploding pain	85	57.4	20	35.7	1.7 (0.9–3.1)	**0.05**
Response to triptans Yes vs. No	102	68.9	36	64.2	0.9 (0.4–1.9)	0.513
Presence of triggers Yes vs. No	71	47.9	24	42.9	0.7 (0.4–1.2)	0.706
Pericranial Muscle tenderness Yes vs. No	79	53.4	26	46.4	0.5 (0.5–1.7)	0.463

p values in bold indicates statistical significance.

Notably, the presence of allodynia showed a marked trend to significance towards association with a clinically meaningful response to fremanezumab (OR: 1.5; 95% CI: 0.6–3.3; $p = 0.071$).

We finally turned to multivariate analysis to identify the independent predictors of adequate response to fremanezumab (only significant variables were included), and we confirmed this independent association only for HFEM (OR of 3.3; 95% CI: 2.3–5.3; $p = 0.02$) coupled with the presence of strict unilateral pain (OR of 2.1; 95% CI: 1.5–4.3; $p = 0.03$) or pain in the ophthalmic trigeminal branch (OR of 2.6; 95% CI: 1.3–7.3; $p = 0.036$).

3.2. Phenotypic Characteristics Comparison between Responders vs. Super-Responders to Fremanezumab

Among a total of 148 responders obtaining an at least 50% reduction in MHD after fremanezumab therapy, 83 responded at 50–74% and 65 at ≥75%, compared to baseline, and were as such classified as either responders or super-responders, respectively. Super-responders more frequently presented allodynia both in univariate (OR of 2.4; 95% CI: 1.2–4.8; $p = 0.022$) and multivariate logistic regression (OR of 2.1; 95% CI: 1.4–6.8; $p = 0.04$) analyses, compared to responders, while all other associations failed to reach significance (Table 3).

Table 3. Incidence of various clinical predictors in migraine patients with response (50–74% reduction in MHD) vs. super-responders (≥75% MHD reduction) to fremanezumab.

Predictors	Responders n = 81		Super-Responders n = 67		O.R (95% CI)	p Value
	N	%	N	%		
Strict unilateral pain	32	39.5	28	41.8	0.7 (0.4–1.4)	0.544
Allodynia	21	25.9	31	46.2	2.4 (1.2–4.8)	**0.022**
Pain in ophthalmic trigeminal branch	18	22.2	12	17.9	0.8 (0.3–1.7)	0.681
Dopaminergic symptoms	48	59.2	37	55.2	0.5 (0.3–1.4)	0.323
Unilateral Autonomic symptoms	33	40.7	23	34.3	0.6 (0.3–1.5)	0.364
Imploding vs. exploding pain	47	58.1	38	56.7	0.8 (0.4–1.7)	0.733
Response to triptans Yes vs. No	59	72.8	43	64.2	1.0 (0.5–2.5)	0.203
Presence of triggers Yes vs. No	38	46.9	33	49.2	0.8 (0.3–1.4)	0.871
Pericranial Muscle tenderness Yes vs. No	44	54.3	35	52.2	0.8 (0.5–1.7)	0.743

p values in bold indicates statistical significance.

4. Discussion

The current post hoc analysis sought to prospectively assess the value of several baseline socio-demographic/clinical parameters or phenotypic profiling in predicting the responders (50–74% response rates) or super-responders (≥75% response rates) to fremanezumab. The main finding to emerge from univariate analyses was that three from the baseline socio-demographic and clinical variables, i.e., age group 41–70 years ($p = 0.02$); female gender ($p = 0.03$); patients with HFEM ($p = 0.001$), and three variables extracted from the phenotypic clinical profile of patients, i.e., strict unilateral pain ($p = 0.05$); pain in the ophthalmic trigeminal branch ($p = 0.04$); and the "imploding" quality of pain ($p = 0.05$), were significantly related to fremanezumab response. However, in multivariate analysis, only HFEM ($p = 0.02$); the presence of strict unilateral rather than alternating pain ($p = 0.03$); and pain location in the ophthalmic trigeminal branch ($p = 0.036$) were independently associated with good response to fremanezumab. Moreover, allodynia ($p = 0.04$) was the only clinical phenotypic variable that was able to positively and independently predict super-responsiveness to fremanezumab.

Our findings, overall, bolster the argument that symptoms related to both peripheral sensitization, i.e., strict unilateral pain and pain location in the ophthalmic trigeminal branch, and also central sensitization, i.e., allodynia, may be associated with good clinical response to fremanezumab. As such, we can assume that its preventive effects are conveyed via the modulation of overactive somatosensory processing and pain thresholds through activation of the trigeminoautonomic reflex [20], while patients with certain migraine phenotypes, characterized by location of pain strictly unilaterally or specifically in the V1 dermatome, may mostly benefit even during the phase of migraine chronification [21]. In addition, it seems that fremanezumab is able to inhibit the sensitization of centrally situated second-order nociceptive neurons [20], and as such patients with allodynia, a feature consistent with central sensitization, may indeed super-respond to fremanezumab [22,23].

Our results are in agreement with previous publications demonstrating that the responsiveness to anti-CGRPs was positively associated with symptoms related to both peripheral and central sensitization [12–14]. The relevance of migraine type, i.e., HFEM over CM, in predicting the therapeutic response to anti-CGRP MAbs has been pointed out also by other research groups, demonstrating that fewer migraine days at baseline was associated with good response [24]. Our findings also partly support the hypothesis that the subjective perception of pain as an "imploding" headache, compared to "exploding" pain, might be a feature with some ability to predict the response to anti-CGRPS; consistent with a similar good response which was previously seen with onabotulinumtoxin-A [25].

However, we were unable to confirm findings from other studies, which favor the role of several other variables in predicting the responsiveness to anti-CGRPs, such as dopaminergic symptoms; autonomic symptoms; absence of psychiatric comorbidities; good response to triptans; normal BMI; age at migraine onset; family history of migraine; number of failed preventive medications; and MIDAS score [12,13,15,24,26–28]. Methodological differences, including populations investigated, sample sizes, and clinical efficacy outcomes studied, may account for discrepancies between results of available studies.

Nonetheless, it should be emphasized that our study comprised a homogenous sample of fremanezumab-treated patients with difficult-to-treat migraine, having at least three previously failed preventive treatments. The latter, in our opinion, should be counted among the strengths of our study, as other relevant publications attempted to identify predictors of response after exposure to mixed antiCGRP MAbs, including erenumab, fremanezumab, and galcanezumab, according to drug market availability or physician's choice [14,29]. In any case, we cannot exclude the presence of other significant predictive socio-demographic or clinical variables than those included in our analysis, and as such a more in-depth clinical profiling may discover other strong predictors of response to fremanezumab.

To explain why we only provide data about predictors of response on no anti-CGRP MAbs for migraine prophylaxis other than fremanezumab, we should mention that fremanezumab was approved first for reimbursement, according to the national policies concerning reimbursement of expensive therapies for migraine (early access release date in late 2020 and formal approval in July 2021) in Greece. Erenumab and galcanezumab received a similar approval quite recently, in February 2022 and in February 2023, respectively. Eptinezumab is currently unavailable in Greece. Both fremanezumab, erenumab and galcanezumab are currently fully reimbursed by the National Health System and social services in Greek patients with HFEM or CM who failed at least three preventive treatments, including OnabotulinumtoxinA in patients clinically classified as having CM [30]. Patients with private insurance that covers the cost of anti-CGRP MAbs also have access to these treatments.

According to international but also national guidelines on the use, monitoring and discontinuation of anti-CGRP MAbs, it is recommended to treat adult patients with 4 or more migraine days per month for at least 3 months before establishing efficacy. With a reduction of >50% in monthly headache days compared to baseline, it is advised to further continue treatment for up to 12–18 months of therapy [19,30,31], and then pause for 1–2 months to monitor for a migraine relapse; in such cases, re-administration of the discontinued anti-CGRP MAb is recommended [19,30,31]. However, in case of 30% of monthly headache days, compared to baseline, after 3 months of therapy, it is advised to continue exposure for another 3 months before concluding on the efficacy of a given anti-CGRP MAb [19,30] Nonetheless, if a reduction of <30% in monthly headache days occurs after 6 months of continuous treatment with the first-line anti-CGRP MAb, it is recommended to switch to another anti-CGRP MAb with different target upon CGRP, i.e., CGRP ligand or CGRP receptor) [32] or to commence dual targeting with onabotulinumtoxinA add-on to anti-CGRP MAb in these treatment-refractory patients [33,34], as a delayed clinically meaningful response is unlikely to occur with further (after 6 months) exposure to initial treatment with the use of either monoclonal antibodies targeting the CGRP ligand or its receptor [35]. A quite recently published report contradicts the latter view, by demonstrating that late responses to anti-CGRP MAbs may occur even beyond 12 months of continuous treatment [36]. Further studies on this clinically important issue are warranted before definite conclusions can be drawn.

5. Conclusions

To conclude from a clinical point of view, our results indicate that a precise phenotypic profiling with identification of pain characteristics consistent with peripheral and/or central sensitization might be able to predict responsiveness to fremanezumab in migraine prophylaxis. Further larger prospective studies, including genetic sequencing and biomarker profiling, are warranted to address the important issue concerning a precise prediction of response to available anti-CGRPs MAbs.

Author Contributions: Conceptualization, A.A.A., E.V.D. and M.V.; methodology, A.A.A., E.V.D., G.X., D.R., P.S., P.L. and M.V.; formal analysis, A.A.A., E.V.D. and M.V.; data curation, A.A.A., E.V.D., G.X., D.R., P.S., P.L. and M.V.; writing—original draft preparation, A.A.A., E.V.D., G.X., D.R., P.S., P.L. and M.V.; writing—review and editing, A.A.A., E.V.D. and M.V.; visualization, A.A.A., E.V.D. and M.V.; supervision, A.A.A., E.V.D. and M.V. All authors have read and agreed to the published version of the manuscript.

Funding: This research received no external funding.

Institutional Review Board Statement: The study was conducted in accordance with the Declaration of Helsinki. The study protocol was approved by the Institutional Review Board of "Agios Andreas" Patras General Hospital.

Informed Consent Statement: Informed consent was obtained from all subjects involved in the study.

Data Availability Statement: The data that support the findings of this study are available from the corresponding author upon reasonable request.

Conflicts of Interest: A.A.A. has received investigator fees and/or advisory board member and/or consultancy and/or travel grants from Allergan-Abbvie, Novartis, and Teva. E.V.D. has received investigator fees and/or advisory board member and/or consultancy and/or travel grants from Allergan-Abbvie, Novartis, Teva, Eli-Lilly, Tikun and Amgen. G.X. has received investigator fees and/or advisory board member and/or consultancy and/or travel grants from Allergan-Abbvie, Teva, UCB, Novartis, ITF Hellas, Innovis. D.R. has received investigator fees and/or advisory board member and/or consultancy and/or travel grants from Allergan-Abbvie, Novartis, and Teva. P.S. has received investigator fees and/or advisory board member and/or consultancy and/or travel grants from Allergan-Abbvie, Novartis, and Teva. P.L. has received investigator fees and/or advisory board member and/or consultancy and/or travel grants from Allergan-Abbvie, and Novartis. M.V. has received investigator fees and/or advisory board member and/or consultancy and/or travel grants from Allergan-Abbvie, Elli- Lilly, Novartis, Teva.

References

1. Wang, X.; Chen, Y.; Song, J.; You, C. Efficacy and Safety of Monoclonal Antibody Against Calcitonin Gene-Related Peptide or Its Receptor for Migraine: A Systematic Review and Network Meta-analysis. *Front. Pharmacol.* **2021**, *12*, 649143. [CrossRef] [PubMed]
2. Deen, M.; Correnti, E.; Kamm, K.; Kelderman, T.; Papetti, L.; Rubio-Beltrán, E.; Vigneri, S.; Edvinsson, L.; Maassen Van Den Brink, A. Blocking CGRP in migraine patients—A review of pros and cons. *J. Headache Pain* **2017**, *18*, 96. [CrossRef]
3. Goadsby, P.J.; Holland, P.R.; Martins-Oliveira, M.; Hoffmann, J.; Schankin, C.; Akerman, S. Pathophysiology of Migraine: A Disorder of Sensory Processing. *Physiol. Rev.* **2017**, *97*, 553–622. [CrossRef]
4. Melo-Carrillo, A.; Strassman, A.M.; Nir, R.-R.; Schain, A.J.; Noseda, R.; Stratton, J.; Burstein, R. Fremanezumab-A Humanized Monoclonal Anti-CGRP Antibody-Inhibits Thinly Myelinated (Aδ) but Not Unmyelinated (C) Meningeal Nociceptors. *J. Neurosci.* **2017**, *37*, 10587–10596. [CrossRef]
5. Silberstein, S.D.; McAllister, P.; Ning, X.; Faulhaber, N.; Lang, N.; Yeung, P.; Schiemann, J.; Aycardi, E.; Cohen, J.M.; Janka, L.; et al. Safety and Tolerability of Fremanezumab for the Prevention of Migraine: A Pooled Analysis of Phases 2b and 3 Clinical Trials. *Headache* **2019**, *59*, 880–890. [CrossRef]
6. Pavelic, A.R.; Wöber, C.; Riederer, F.; Zebenholzer, K. Monoclonal Antibodies against Calcitonin Gene-Related Peptide for Migraine Prophylaxis: A Systematic Review of Real-World Data. *Cells* **2022**, *12*, 143. [CrossRef]
7. Murray, A.M.; Stern, J.I.; Robertson, C.E.; Chiang, C.C. Real-World Patient Experience of CGRP-Targeting Therapy for Migraine: A Narrative Review. *Curr. Pain Headache Rep.* **2022**, *26*, 783–794. [CrossRef]
8. Vandervorst, F.; Van Deun, L.; Van Dycke, A.; Paemeleire, K.; Reuter, U.; Schoenen, J.; Versijpt, J. CGRP monoclonal antibodies in migraine: An efficacy and tolerability comparison with standard prophylactic drugs. *J. Headache Pain* **2021**, *22*, 128. [CrossRef]

9. Argyriou, A.A.; Dermitzakis, E.V.; Xiromerisiou, G.; Rallis, D.; Soldatos, P.; Litsardopoulos, P.; Vikelis, M. Efficacy and safety of fremanezumab for migraine prophylaxis in patients with at least three previous preventive failures: Prospective, multicenter, real-world data from a Greek registry. *Eur. J. Neurol.* **2023**, *30*, 1435–1442. [CrossRef]
10. Messina, R.; Huessler, E.M.; Puledda, F.; Haghdoost, F.; Lebedeva, E.R.; Diener, H.C. Safety and tolerability of monoclonal antibodies targeting the CGRP pathway and gepants in migraine prevention: A systematic review and network meta-analysis. *Cephalalgia* **2023**, *43*, 3331024231152169. [CrossRef]
11. Ashina, M.; Terwindt, G.M.; Al-Karagholi, M.A.-M.; de Boer, I.; Lee, M.J.; Hay, D.L.; Schulte, L.H.; Hadjikhani, N.; Sinclair, A.J.; Ashina, H.; et al. Migraine: Disease characterisation, biomarkers, and precision medicine. *Lancet* **2021**, *397*, 1496–1504. [CrossRef] [PubMed]
12. Barbanti, P.; Aurilia, C.; Egeo, G.; Fofi, L.; Cevoli, S.; Colombo, B.; Filippi, M.; Frediani, F.; Bono, F.; Grazzi, L.; et al. Erenumab in the prevention of high-frequency episodic and chronic migraine: Erenumab in Real Life in Italy (EARLY), the first Italian multicenter, prospective real-life study. *Headache* **2021**, *61*, 363–372. [CrossRef] [PubMed]
13. Vernieri, F.; Altamura, C.; Brunelli, N.; Costa, C.M.; Aurilia, C.; Egeo, G.; Fofi, L.; Favoni, V.; Pierangeli, G.; Lovati, C.; et al. Galcanezumab for the prevention of high frequency episodic and chronic migraine in real life in Italy: A multicenter prospective cohort study (the GARLIT study). *J. Headache Pain* **2021**, *22*, 35. [CrossRef] [PubMed]
14. Barbanti, P.; Egeo, G.; Aurilia, C.; Altamura, C.; d'Onofrio, F.; Finocchi, C.; Albanese, M.; Aguggia, M.; Rao, R.; Zucco, M.; et al. Predictors of response to anti-CGRP monoclonal antibodies: A 24-week, multicenter, prospective study on 864 migraine patients. *J. Headache Pain* **2022**, *23*, 138. [CrossRef]
15. Nowaczewska, M.; Straburzyński, M.; Waliszewska-Prosół, M.; Meder, G.; Janiak-Kiszka, J.; Kaźmierczak, W. Cerebral Blood Flow and Other Predictors of Responsiveness to Erenumab and Fremanezumab in Migraine-A Real-Life Study. *Front. Neurol.* **2022**, *13*, 895476. [CrossRef] [PubMed]
16. Arnold, M. Headache Classification Committee of the International Headache Society (IHS) the International Classification of Headache Disorders, 3rd edition. *Cephalalgia* **2018**, *38*, 1–211.
17. Teva Pharmaceuticals USA, Inc. Highlights for Prescribing Information. AJOVY TM (Fremanezumab-Vfrm) Injection, for Subcutaneous Use. Initial. U.S. 2018. Available online: https://www.accessdata.fda.gov/drugsatfda_docs/label/2018/761089s000lbl.pdf (accessed on 15 February 2023).
18. Barbanti, P.; Aurilia, C.; Dall'Armi, V.; Egeo, G.; Fofi, L.; Bonassi, S. The phenotype of migraine with unilateral cranial autonomic symptoms documents increased peripheral and central trigeminal sensitization. A case series of 757 patients. *Cephalalgia* **2016**, *36*, 1334–1340. [CrossRef]
19. Sacco, S.; Bendtsen, L.; Ashina, M.; Reuter, U.; Terwindt, G.; Mitsikostas, D.D.; Martelletti, P. European headache federation guideline on the use of monoclonal antibodies acting on the calcitonin gene related peptide or its receptor for migraine prevention. *J. Headache Pain* **2019**, *20*, 6. [CrossRef]
20. Barbanti, P.; Egeo, G.; Mitsikostas, D.D. Trigeminal-Targeted Treatments in Migraine: Is 60% the Magic Number? *Headache* **2019**, *59*, 1659–1661. [CrossRef]
21. Domínguez, C.; Pozo-Rosich, P.; Leira, Y.; Leira, R. Unilateral pain and shorter duration of chronic migraine are significant predictors of response to onabotulinumtoxin A. *Eur. J. Neurol.* **2018**, *25*, e48. [CrossRef]
22. Iyengar, S.; Ossipov, M.H.; Johnson, K.W. The role of calcitonin gene-related peptide in peripheral and central pain mechanisms including migraine. *Pain* **2017**, *158*, 543–559. [CrossRef] [PubMed]
23. Hargreaves, R.; Olesen, J. Calcitonin Gene-Related Peptide Modulators—The History and Renaissance of a New Migraine Drug Class. *Headache* **2019**, *59*, 951–970. [CrossRef]
24. Iannone, L.F.; Fattori, D.; Benemei, S.; Chiarugi, A.; Geppetti, P.; De Cesaris, F. Long-Term Effectiveness of Three Anti-CGRP Monoclonal Antibodies in Resistant Chronic Migraine Patients Based on the MIDAS score. *CNS Drugs* **2022**, *36*, 191–202. [CrossRef]
25. Jakubowski, M.; McAllister, P.J.; Bajwa, Z.H.; Ward, T.N.; Smith, P.; Burstein, R. Exploding vs. imploding headache in migraine prophylaxis with Botulinum Toxin A. *Pain* **2006**, *125*, 286–295. [CrossRef]
26. Zecca, C.; Cargnin, S.; Schankin, C.; Giannantoni, N.M.; Viana, M.; Maraffi, I.; Riccitelli, G.C.; Sihabdeen, S.; Terrazzino, S.; Gobbi, C. Clinic and genetic predictors in response to erenumab. *Eur. J. Neurol.* **2022**, *29*, 1209–1217. [CrossRef]
27. Frattale, I.; Caponnetto, V.; Casalena, A.; Assetta, M.; Maddestra, M.; Marzoli, F.; Affaitati, G.; Giamberardino, M.A.; Viola, S.; Gabriele, A.; et al. Association between response to triptans and response to erenumab: Real-life data. *J. Headache Pain* **2021**, *22*, 1. [CrossRef]
28. Salem-Abdou, H.; Simonyan, D.; Puymirat, J. Identification of predictors of response to Erenumab in a cohort of patients with migraine. *Cephalalgia Rep.* **2021**, *4*, 25158163211026646. [CrossRef]
29. Caronna, E.; Gallardo, V.J.; Alpuente, A.; Torres-Ferrus, M.; Pozo-Rosich, P. Anti-CGRP monoclonal antibodies in chronic migraine with medication overuse: Real-life effectiveness and predictors of response at 6 months. *J. Headache Pain* **2021**, *22*, 120. [CrossRef]
30. Vikelis, M.; Dermitzakis, E.V.; Argyriou, A.A.; Rikos, D.; Soldatos, P.; Vlachos, G.S.; Notas, K.; Rudolf, J.; Dardiotis, E.; Karapanayiotides, T.; et al. Consensus article: The opinion of the headache scientific panel of the Hellenic Neurological Society on the use of monoclonal antibodies and small molecules targeting the CGRP pathway in the treatment of migraine and cluster headache in clinical practice. *Arch. Clin. Neurol.* **2023**, *31*, 18.

31. Al-Hassany, L.; Lyons, H.S.; Boucherie, D.M.; Farham, F.; Lange, K.S.; Marschollek, K.; Onan, D.; Pensato, U.; Storch, E.; Torrente, A.; et al. The sense of stopping migraine prophylaxis. *J. Headache Pain* **2023**, *24*, 9. [CrossRef]
32. Overeem, L.H.; Peikert, A.; Hofacker, M.D.; Kamm, K.; Ruscheweyh, R.; Gendolla, A.; Raffaelli, B.; Reuter, U.; Neeb, L. Effect of antibody switch in non-responders to a CGRP receptor antibody treatment in migraine: A multi-center retrospective cohort study. *Cephalalgia* **2022**, *42*, 291–301. [CrossRef]
33. Scuteri, D.; Tonin, P.; Nicotera, P.; Vulnera, M.; Altieri, G.C.; Tarsitano, A.; Bagetta, G.; Corasaniti, M.T. Pooled Analysis of Real-World Evidence Supports Anti-CGRP mAbs and OnabotulinumtoxinA Combined Trial in Chronic Migraine. *Toxins* **2022**, *14*, 529. [CrossRef]
34. Argyriou, A.A.; Dermitzakis, E.V.; Xiromerisiou, G.; Vikelis, M. OnabotulinumtoxinA Add-On to Monoclonal Anti-CGRP Antibodies in Treatment-Refractory Chronic Migraine. *Toxins* **2022**, *14*, 847. [CrossRef]
35. Andreou, A.P.; Fuccaro, M.; Hill, B.; Murphy, M.; Caponnetto, V.; Kilner, R.; Lambru, G. Two-year effectiveness of erenumab in resistant chronic migraine: A prospective real-world analysis. *J. Headache Pain* **2022**, *23*, 139. [CrossRef]
36. Barbanti, P.; Aurilia, C.; Egeo, G.; Torelli, P.; Proietti, S.; Cevoli, S.; Bonassi, S.; Italian Migraine Registry study group. Late Response to Anti-CGRP Monoclonal Antibodies in Migraine: A Multicenter, Prospective, Observational Study. *Neurology* **2023**. *ahead of print*. [CrossRef]

Disclaimer/Publisher's Note: The statements, opinions and data contained in all publications are solely those of the individual author(s) and contributor(s) and not of MDPI and/or the editor(s). MDPI and/or the editor(s) disclaim responsibility for any injury to people or property resulting from any ideas, methods, instructions or products referred to in the content.

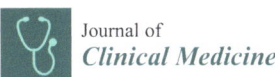

Article

Effects of Fremanezumab on Psychiatric Comorbidities in Difficult-to-Treat Patients with Chronic Migraine: Post Hoc Analysis of a Prospective, Multicenter, Real-World Greek Registry

Michail Vikelis [1,*,†], Emmanouil V. Dermitzakis [2,†], Georgia Xiromerisiou [3], Dimitrios Rallis [4], Panagiotis Soldatos [5], Pantelis Litsardopoulos [6], Dimitrios Rikos [7] and Andreas A. Argyriou [6]

1. Headache Clinic, Mediterraneo Hospital, 16675 Athens, Greece
2. Euromedica General Clinic, 54645 Thessaloniki, Greece; manolis.dermitzakis@gmail.com
3. Department of Neurology, University Hospital of Larissa, University of Thessaly, 41110 Larissa, Greece; georgiaxiromerisiou@gmail.com
4. Department of Neurology, Tzaneio General Hospital of Piraeus, 18536 Athens, Greece; jimrallis@hotmail.com
5. Independent Researcher, 24100 Kalamata, Greece; soldatosp@gmail.com
6. Headache Outpatient Clinic, Department of Neurology, Agios Andreas State General Hospital of Patras, 26335 Patras, Greece; pantelis84@hotmail.com (P.L.); andargyriou@yahoo.gr (A.A.A.)
7. 404 Military Hospital, 41222 Larisa, Greece; rikosd@hotmail.com
* Correspondence: mvikelis@headaches.gr
† These authors contributed equally to this work.

Abstract: Objective: this post hoc analysis aimed to evaluate the efficacy of fremanezumab in difficult-to-treat chronic migraine (CM) patients with and without psychiatric comorbidities (PCs), mainly anxiety and/or depression. Methods: We assessed data from CM patients with and without PCs who failed at least 3 preventives and eventually received at least 3 consecutive monthly doses of fremanezumab 225 mg. Outcomes included the crude response ($\geq$50% reduction in monthly headache days (MHDs)) rates to fremanezumab from the baseline to the last clinical follow-up. The changes in MHDs; MHDs of moderate/greater severity; monthly days with intake of abortive medication; and the proportion of patients' changing status from with PCs to decreased/without PCs were also compared. Disability and quality of life (QOL) outcomes were also assessed. Results: Of 107 patients enrolled, 65 (60.7%) had baseline PCs. The percentage of patients with (n = 38/65; 58.5%) and without (n = 28/42; 66.6%) PCs that achieved a $\geq$50% reduction in MHDs with fremanezumab was comparable (p = 0.41), whereas MHDs were significantly reduced (difference vs. baseline) in both patients with PCs (mean −8.9 (standard error: 6.8); p < 0.001) and without PCs (−9.8 (7.5); p < 0.001). Both groups experienced significant improvements in all other efficacy, disability, and QOL outcomes at comparable rates, including in MHD reduction. A significant proportion of fremanezumab-treated patients with baseline PCs de-escalated in corresponding severities or even reverted to no PCs (28/65; 43.1%) post-fremanezumab. Conclusions: fremanezumab appears to be effective as a preventive treatment in difficult-to-treat CM patients with and without PCs while also being beneficial in reducing the severity of comorbid anxiety and/or depression.

Keywords: CGRP; monoclonal antibodies; chronic migraine; fremanezumab; psychiatric comorbidities; efficacy; response

1. Introduction

Migraine ranks among the most common primary headache disorders. It is characterized by attacks of headache and associated symptoms, including nausea, vomiting, photophobia, or phonophobia. Most patients suffer from episodic migraine (EM) and experience migraine attacks on less than 15 days per month. However, up to 6% of individuals with EM progress to chronic migraine (CM), defined as headaches occurring on 15 or more days per month, with migrainous features or a response to migraine-specific medications for at least 8 days per month. Chronic migraine can be with or without aura, and although there is a requirement for symptoms to be present for three months in order to diagnose it, most patients experience it for years before being diagnosed. A sizable proportion of CM patients experience severe headaches almost daily, resulting in the generation of considerable disability, a deterioration in their quality of life, and evidence of clinically significant psychological distress [1].

Migraine and psychiatric disorders, mainly depression and/or anxiety, are frequently comorbid in CM, with a lifetime prevalence of depression significantly above the corresponding prevalence seen in controls without migraine [2] or even in EM patients [3]. Moreover, a bidirectional association between psychiatric comorbidities (PCs) and migraine has been identified, as the frequency of monthly headache days (MHDs) proportionally increases with the frequency and severity of PCs. Thus, the comorbid depression and/or anxiety significantly contributes to increasing the risk of progression from EM to CM [4].

A number of non-specific medications (e.g., beta blockers, anticonvulsants, and antidepressants) have long been used for migraine prevention; however, clinical experience has shown that both the efficacy and safety/tolerability of these medications is rather modest, and there is a need for optimized and specific migraine-preventive medications, rather than the current standard of care with the use of oral preventatives, such as topiramate [5,6]. The recognition of calcitonin gene-related peptide (CGRP) as a neuropeptide critically involved in both central and peripheral (neuronal, sensitization, vasodilation, inflammation, and protein extravasation) processes underlying the pathophysiology of migraine has revolutionized the prophylactic treatment of migraine [7]. Several clinical studies have shown that targeted therapies with the use of anti-CGRP monoclonal antibodies (anti-CGRP MAbs) were efficacious and safe in the prophylaxis of both EM and CM [8,9].

Fremanezumab is a fully humanized IgG 2 (delta) a/kappa monoclonal antibody that was approved in September 2018 in the United States and in January 2019 by the EMA/CHMP for the prophylactic treatment of both EM and CM, based on its ability to potently and selectively bind to both CGRP isoforms (α- and β-CGRP), preventing them from binding to the CGRP receptor in the trigeminal ganglion and meningeal nociceptors in order to selectively inhibit the activation of the trigeminovascular pain pathway [10–12]. Subsequently, the excellent efficacy/safety profile of fremanezumab in migraine prophylaxis was documented in several real-world studies [9,13].

Post hoc analyses of data from the HALO CM study demonstrated significant reductions in MHDs in patients with comorbid depression, significant reductions in disability, and significant improvements in QOL outcomes. Additionally, a significant proportion of patients with evidence of baseline major depressive symptomatology experienced 50% reductions in severities, as assessed by the PHQ-9 scale, over the study period while treated with fremanezumab, thus providing evidence for the possibility of improvements in both migraine and depression [14].

Fremanezumab received market authorization in Greece for migraine prevention in 2020 and was granted a positive opinion from the national insurance organization (EOPPY) in 2021 to be fully reimbursed in patients suffering from high-frequency EM (HFEM: 8–14 days/month) who previously failed to first-line treatments. CM reimbursement additionally requires failure to onabotulinumtoxinA. We have recently demonstrated in real-world conditions that fremanezumab was able to be effective and safe when administered for migraine prophylaxis in difficult-to-treat migraine patients with either HFEM or CM [15]. We subsequently reported that a precise phenotypic profiling with the identification of pain characteristics consistent with peripheral and/or central sensitization might reliably predict the responsiveness to fremanezumab [16]. In the latter post hoc analysis, the baseline occurrence of PCs was not found to be associated with response to fremanezumab, and patients responded equally regardless of comorbid PCs [16].

To specifically test the latter clinical scenario in a homogenous cohort of CM patients, the aim of this post hoc analysis of data extracted from a prospective, multicenter, Greek registry was to evaluate the efficacy of fremanezumab in difficult-to-treat CM patients with and without PCs, mainly anxiety and/or depression.

2. Materials and Methods

The study was conducted in accordance with the requirements of the Declaration of Helsinki, the protocol was approved by the Institutional Review Board of "Agios Andreas" Patras General Hospital, and each patient provided an informed consent before entering the study. In this post-hoc analysis of data extracted from a prospective, observational study, the study population was composed of male or female patients, aged 18 years and older, diagnosed with CM with or without medication-overuse headache (MOH), who were prescribed fremanezumab as a treatment decision of their physician before enrollment in this study. Fremanezumab treatment was commenced strictly in line with the approved indication as described in the Summary of Product Characteristics (SmPC) [17] and current national reimbursement policies. These policies dictate that full reimbursement of fremanezumab is granted in CM patients who inadequately responded or were intolerant to first-line oral treatments and onabotulinumtoxinA, given quarterly for 3 consecutive courses [18,19].

Eligibility was confirmed by a protocol-specific checklist. Adult patients were included in the study only if all of the following criteria were met: (i) the patient had read and signed the informed consent after receiving all information about the study; (ii) the patient had a formal diagnosis of CM, according to the international diagnostic criteria [20]; (iii) the patient has been prescribed fremanezumab as a treatment decision of their physician, according to the SmPC [17]; (iv) the patient was naïve to prior exposure with anti-CGRP MAbs; (v) the patient had been maintaining a daily headache diary as part of their routine disease management and had maintained the diary for at least 21 days in the 28 days prior to fremanezumab treatment initiation for 2 consecutive months; (vi) the patient's headache diary ideally captured information on headache duration, headache severity, headache characteristics, and days with intake of any acute medication for headache relief; (vii) the patient was able to understand and was willing to keep records in the paper headache diary for the course of the study. Exclusion criteria included any contraindication to fremanezumab, according to the standard clinical practice and the approved SmPC [17]. Patients participating in any interventional clinical trial in CM, patients who were pregnant, or patients who were nursing females were excluded. Moreover, patients with major psychiatric disorder, such as autism, uncontrolled bipolar disorder, and schizophrenia, were also excluded from participating in this study.

Fremanezumab (Ajovy® 225mg/pf-syr, Teva Pharma, Athens-Greece) was prescribed either as 225 mg monthly (every 28–30 days) or 675 mg quarterly (every 90 days), depending on the decision of the patient's physician and standards of care. Patients were guided by their treating physician to use their fremanezumab solution for self-injection, as described in the SmPC, for at least 3 months (12 weeks) before establishing efficacy. The end of the observational period was defined as the last routine clinic visit during the observational period of each patient. Hence, patients in this group were followed for 3–18 months of fremanezumab exposure.

Effectiveness data were evaluated using the information recorded by patient-reported outcome measures in the patients' diaries in paper format (headache diary compliance was set to at least 80% of total days) and from validated headache-related disability tools, including questionnaires, used in real-world clinical practice. The primary endpoint was to evaluate the mean change from baseline in the monthly average number of migraine days (MHDs) at the last routine follow-up, whereas the secondary endpoints for effectiveness were the following: (i) the proportion of patients reaching at least 50% reduction in the mean MHDs during the clinical follow-up period (>3 months) after the first dose of fremanezumab; (ii) the change in mean MHDs with peak moderate/severe headache intensity, i.e., more than 4 out of 10 on a 0–10 numerical scale; (iii) the change in mean monthly days with consumption of any abortive headache medications; (iv) the documentation of changes in disability score, as measured by the Migraine Disability Assessment (MIDAS) questionnaire [21], and also in the headache-related disability score, as measured by the 6-item headache impact test (HIT-6) [22] and quality of life assessment, as assessed by the EQ-5D questionnaire [23]. EQ-5D is composed of a "self-classifier" part and a thermometer-like vertical Visual Analog Scale (VAS), by which respondents can self-rate their perceived health status with a grade ranging from 0 to 100, with higher scores indicative of higher health status [23]. The incidence and severity of psychological distress at baseline to document PCs was assessed using the HADS [24] scale, consisting of 14 items: 7 for anxiety (HADS-A) and 7 for depression (HADS-D). All items are based solely on the psychological symptoms of mood and anxiety disorders to the exclusion of somatic symptoms. Each subscale is scored from 0 to 21, with scores of 0–7 representing a non-case of anxiety and depression, 8–10 a doubtful or borderline case, and 11–21 a definite case.

Finally, the patients' perception of the impact of fremanezumab treatment on disease management and satisfaction was evaluated with the use of the 7-point (1 stands for "no change" and 7 for "considerable improvement") self-report "Patient Global Impression of Change" (PGIC) questionnaire [25]. The cut-off score to define a "clinically significant benefit" was set to a PGIC score of ≥ 5, according to the IMMPACT recommendations [26].

Statistical Analysis

Descriptive statistics were generated for all variables. Two-sided chi-squared tests were used to compare categorical data between patients with baseline PCs vs. those without PCs. For within-group comparisons, the paired-samples t-test was used to reveal any potential changes in mean headache outcome scores from baseline to post-fremanezumab follow-up. For between-group comparisons, the changes in mean headache outcome scores were evaluated by subtracting each patient's baseline value from her/his last value and were calculated with the use of the independent-sample t-tests. Unless otherwise stated, all tests were two-sided, and significance was set at $p < 0.05$. Statistics were performed by employing the SPSS for Windows (release 27.0; SPSS Inc., Chicago, IL, USA).

3. Results

The study sample consisted of 14 males (13.1%) and 93 females (86.9%) with a mean age of 49.8 ± 10.7 (range: 23–70) years. Of 107 patients enrolled, 65 (60.7%) had baseline PCs. The majority of them ($n = 37$; 56.9%) had a normal BMI of <24.9 and were diagnosed with concurrent MOH ($n = 61$; 93.8%). Among PCs, mixed anxiety and depression disorders were most commonly seen ($n = 26$; 40%), followed by anxiety disorders ($n = 24$; 36.9%), depression ($n = 13$; 20%), and bipolar disorders ($n = 2$; 3.1%). These patients were treated with venlafaxine ($n = 22$), duloxetine ($n = 10$), amitriptyline ($n = 24$), and other SSRIs ($n = 9$). The overall baseline epidemiological and clinical characteristics of participants, according to whether they had PCs or not at baseline, are described in Table 1.

3.1. Within-Group Comparison of Fremanezumab-Related Efficacy Headache Outcomes, according to Baseline Evidence or Lack of Psychiatric Comorbidities

3.1.1. Fremanezumab-Treated Patients without Baseline PCs ($n = 42$)

MHDs were significantly reduced (difference vs. baseline) in patients without PCs (22.4 ± 5.0 vs. 12.6 ± 7.6; $p < 0.001$). Likewise, there was a significant decrease in MHDs with moderate/severe headache (more than 4/10 in VAS) compared with the baseline (16.8 ± 6.5 vs. 9.7 ± 7.7; $p < 0.001$), whereas the number of monthly days with intake of acute headache medications was also significantly lower (18.9 ± 6.6 vs. 10.5 ± 7.3; $p < 0.001$).

A total of 28/42 (66.6%) patients had $\geq 50\%$ reduction in MHDs with fremanezumab and were as such defined as treatment responders. Among them, 17 and 11 patients successfully achieved response at 50% and 75%, respectively, after treatment with fremanezumab. As expected, the efficacy to therapy influenced the disability and QOL outcomes. MIDAS (113.4 ± 69.3 vs. 54.6 ± 52.6; $p = 0.018$) and HIT-6 (67.4 ± 8.4 vs. 59.5 ± 10.5; $p = 0.025$)

scores decreased, and the EQ5D scores (46.6 ± 19.3 vs. 68.5 ± 20.3; $p = 0.05$) increased. All 28 treatment responders in this group remained satisfied to score ≥5 on PGIC; specifically, 7 scored 5, 18 scored 6, and 3 scored 7 on PGIC.

Table 1. Demographic and clinical characteristics of fremanezumab-treated CM patients with and without PCs.

Variable Participants n = 107	Patients without PCs n = 42 n %	Patients with PCs n = 65 n %
Gender		
Females	34 80.9	59 90.8
Males	8 19.1	6 9.2
Age ± SD (range)	49.6 ± 10.1 (26–70)	50.1 ± 11.1 (23–70)
Number of previously used preventative medications		
Median value (range)	5 (3–7)	5 (3–8)
Years ± SD (range) with chronic migraine	29.8 ± 9.9 (12–41)	28.0 ± 9.6 (7–45)
Body mass index status		
Normal (18–24.9)	22 52.4	37 56.9
Overweight (25–29.9)	17 40.5	18 27.7
Obese (>30)	3 7.1	10 15.4
Psychiatric comorbidities	0 0	65 100
Anxiety disorder	0	24
Depression	0	13
Mixed anxiety and depression disorder	0	26
Bipolar disorder (stable—in remission)	0	2
Medication-overuse headache		
Yes	37 88.1	61 93.8
No	5 11.9	4 6.2

3.1.2. Fremanezumab-Treated Patients with Baseline PCs (*n* = 65)

Comparably to patients without PCs, participants with evidence of psychopathology experienced a significant decrease in MHDs between the baseline and last efficacy follow-up (23.9 ± 5.0 vs. 14.1 ± 7.8; $p < 0.001$). Likewise, there was a significant decrease in the number of MHDs with peak headache intensity of ≥5 (17.3 ± 5.1 vs. 10.4 ± 6.4; $p < 0.001$) and also in monthly days with intake of acute headache medications (21.8 ± 6.1 vs. 12.8 ± 7.9; $p < 0.001$). A total of 38/65 (58.5%) patients were classified as responders as they achieved a ≥50% decrease in MHDs with fremanezumab: 23 at 50% and 15 at 75%. The changes in disability and QOL outcomes clearly favored fremanezumab treatment, which was demonstrated by the reduced MIDAS (111.4 ± 58.7 vs. 67.5 ± 54.4; $p = 0.002$) and HIT-6 (70.0 ± 7.4 vs. 61.6 ± 11.2; $p < 0.001$) scores and a strong tendency of significantly higher EQ5D scores (45.9 ± 20.5 vs. 62.9 ± 22.7; $p = 0.08$). All 38 treatment responders in this group were satisfied with fremanezumab treatment and scored ≥5 on PGIC; specifically, 12 scored 5, 24 scored 6, and 2 scored 7 on PGIC. Finally, a significant proportion of fremanezumab-treated patients with baseline PCs de-escalated in corresponding severities or even reverted to no PCs (28/65; 43.1%) post-fremanezumab. In support of the latter finding, there were improvements in both HADS-A (13.4 ± 4.1 vs. 11.1 ± 4.1; $p < 0.001$) and HADS-D scores (11.9 ± 4.6 vs. 10.2 ± 3.5; $p < 0.001$) post-fremanezumab, compared with the baseline. The improvements in PC severities persisted throughout the study period.

3.2. Between-Group Comparison of Fremanezumab-Related Efficacy Headache Outcomes, according to Baseline Evidence or Lack of Psychiatric Comorbidities

Both groups experienced significant improvements in all efficacy, disability, and QOL outcomes at comparable rates, including in MHD reduction. Figure 1 shows the between-group changes in all fremanezumab-related efficacy headache outcomes, compared with the baseline, in CM patients with and without PCs.

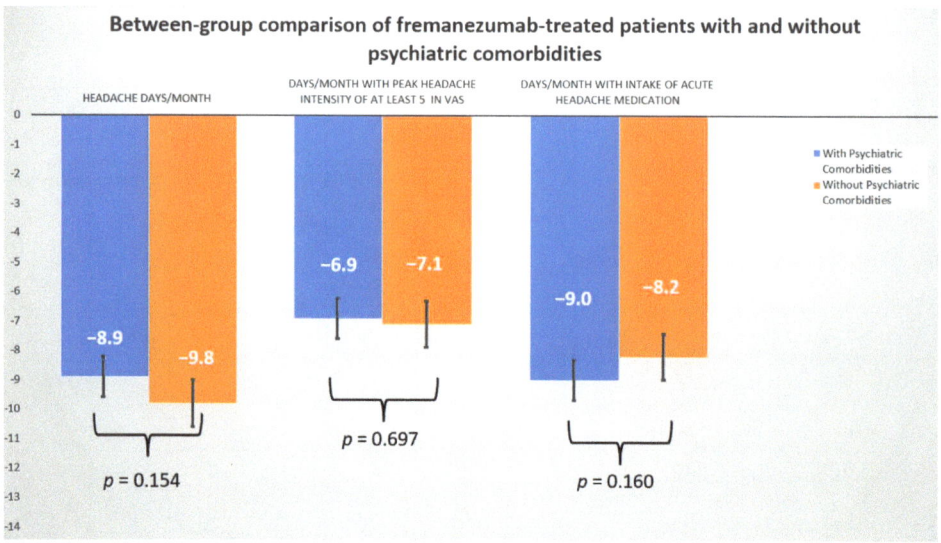

Figure 1. Changes in mean fremanezumab-related headache efficacy scores from baseline to the last follow-up between treatment groups.

Likewise, as depicted in Figure 2, the number of treatment responders with a ≥50% reduction in MHDs with fremanezumab was similar ($p = 0.41$) between patients with ($n = 38/65$; 58.5%) and without ($n = 28/42$; 66.6%) PCs.

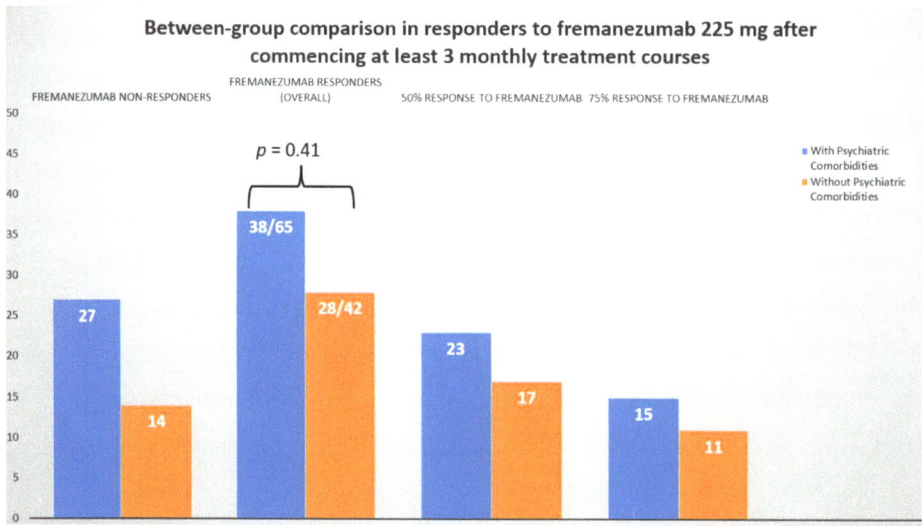

Figure 2. Differences in the number of fremanezumab responders at the last follow-up compared with baseline MHDs between patients with vs. without PCs.

4. Discussion

The current post hoc analysis sought to prospectively assess the efficacy of fremanezumab in CM patients with and without PCs in order to guide better treatment decisions by providing real-world evidence of outcomes with fremanezumab treatment in a homogenous cohort of CM patients with and without PCs, mainly anxiety and/or depression. Our main finding to emerge was that both CM patients with and without PCs comparably benefited from fremanezumab with significant reductions in MHDs and disability and an improvement in their QOL, while improvements in the severities of baseline PCs can also be anticipated during the course of treatment in about 45% of patients.

Our results are in agreement with previous findings from real-world studies demonstrating that fremanezumab was able to exert sustained reductions in MHDs across subgroups of migraine patients with comorbid anxiety and/or depression, whereas improvements in the severities of PCs might also occur in up to 50% of treated patients [27], with reductions in the number of patients who were prescribed antidepressants or anxiolytic medications [28]. These real-world data taken together, including ours, are supportive of the findings from post hoc analyses of data from the HALO CM study demonstrating that CM patients with comorbid depression and a baseline PHQ-9 score of 10 to 19, consistent with moderate-to-severe depression, experienced reductions in PHQ-9 of 9.5 to 10.5 points on average over the 12 weeks of the study when treated with fremanezumab [14]. Moreover, the results of a post hoc analysis pooling the results of two phase-three EM studies on the efficacy of another anti-CGRP MAb, i.e., galcanezumab, targeting the CGRP ligand (same as fremanezumab) for the prevention of migraine in patients with and without comorbid anxiety and/or depression showed that a comorbid medical history of anxiety and/or depression at baseline does not seem to interfere with the response to galcanezumab, and patients comparably respond regardless of their psychiatric history [29].

A possible shared pathogenesis of migraine and PCs with distinct pathophysiological mechanisms, overlapping or interacting with each other, has been previously suggested. However, it remains unclear whether migraine is caused by or is the cause of PCs. Hence, anxiety and/or depression may be able to trigger migraine attacks, while patients with frequent and severe MHDs, such as those suffering from CM, have increased susceptibility to be psychologically distressed. Shared genetic factors with evidence of a significant genetic overlap in identified loci (three SNPs: rs146377178, rs672931, and rs11858956 and two genes: ANKDD1B and KCNK5) for migraine and major depressive disorder might also cause the response in the bidirectional association between these medical conditions [30,31].

Nonetheless, neurochemical alterations—consisting of altered endocannabinoid and serum serotonin levels, which increase during migraine attacks and decrease in between them [32–34], coupled with decreased GABA cerebrospinal fluid levels in CM patients with comorbid depression [35]—may play a key role in the pathophysiology of such a psychiatric bidirectional comorbidity with migraine. Specifically, this serotoninergic imbalance has been suggested to alter the activity of the brainstem nuclei; enhance the activation of the trigeminovascular nociceptive pathway; and possibly also facilitate the generation of cortical spreading depression [36]. In accordance with the latter theory, medications acting on the serotoninergic system, including tricyclic antidepressants, and selective serotonin noradrenaline reuptake inhibitors are prescribed to patients for both EM and CM prophylaxis [37]. Moreover, dysregulation (hyperactivation) of the hypothalamic–pituitary–adrenal axis; estrogen and progesterone influence affecting the vascular endothelium and pain processing systems; neuroinflammation with elevated serum levels of inflammatory markers; and psychological factors, such as stress and sleep deprivation have been suggested to be involved in the intrinsic relationships between migraine and PCs [38–40]. Shared environmental factors and obesity might also contribute to the development of both migraine and comorbid depression and/or anxiety [41].

Finally, CGRP receptors are also implicated in the neurochemical alterations underlying a shared pathophysiology between migraine and PCs via their activation in the bed nucleus of the stria terminalis, strongly suggesting that the inhibition of CGRP receptors with the use of anti-CGRP MAbs may be a clinically useful strategy to achieve likely reductions in both migraine and PC severities [42]. From a clinical point of view, the involvement of CGRP in the pathophysiology of generalized anxiety disorder and possibly in depression might explain the dual beneficial effect of fremanezumab in reducing the severities of both migraine and PCs, as thoroughly demonstrated in this study.

It should be noted that our study, being a post hoc analysis, was not specifically designed to compare the two groups, namely, those with and without PCs, and this should be acknowledged as a limitation preventing the generalizability of our findings. In addition, our sample size was not very large, and this fact should also be noted as a limitation of the study. Nonetheless, our study included a homogenous sample of 107 fremanezumab-treated CM patients with difficult-to-treat migraine, who were studied with quantitative efficacy outcomes and with qualitative patient-reported tools for disability and QOL, and this thorough assessment should be counted among its strengths. Lastly, HADS represents an internationally acceptable instrument for rating psychological morbidity in migraine patients [43–45].

5. Conclusions

To conclude from a clinical point of view, our results indicate that fremanezumab appears to be effective as a preventive treatment in difficult-to-treat CM patients with or without PCs while also being beneficial in reducing the severity of comorbid anxiety and/or depression. The demonstrated efficacy, favorable safety, and tolerability of fremanezumab indicate its substantial therapeutic potential for patients with CM and comorbid PCs. Further studies specifically designed to compare PC subgroups and assess the changes in the severities of psychiatric symptoms over time with fremanezumab treatment are warranted. Towards meeting the latter need, the results of the ongoing UNITE study are anticipated [46] to further shed light on this clinically important issue.

Author Contributions: Conceptualization, M.V., E.V.D. and A.A.A.; methodology, M.V., E.V.D., G.X., D.R. (Dimitrios Rallis), P.S., P.L., D.R. (Dimitrios Rikos) and A.A.A.; formal analysis, M.V., E.V.D. and A.A.A.; data curation, M.V., E.V.D., G.X., D.R. (Dimitrios Rallis), P.S., P.L. and A.A.A.; writing—original draft preparation, M.V., E.V.D., G.X., D.R. (Dimitrios Rallis), P.S., P.L., D.R. (Dimitrios Rikos) and A.A.A.; writing—review and editing, M.V., E.V.D. and A.A.A.; visualization, M.V. and E.V.D.; supervision, M.V., E.V.D. and A.A.A. All authors have read and agreed to the published version of the manuscript.

Funding: M.V. has received investigator fees and/or advisory board member and/or consultancy and/or travel grants from Allergan-Abbvie, Elli-Lilly, Novartis, Teva, Lundbeck, and Pfizer. E.V.D. has received investigator fees and/or advisory board member and/or consultancy and/or travel grants from Allergan-Abbvie, Novartis, Teva, Eli-Lilly, Tikun, Lundbeck, and Pfizer. G.X. has received investigator fees and/or advisory board member and/or consultancy and/or travel grants from Allergan-Abbvie, Teva, UCB, Novartis, ITF Hellas, and Innovis. D.R. (Dimitrios Rallis) has received investigator fees and/or advisory board member and/or consultancy and/or travel grants from Allergan-Abbvie, Novartis, and Teva. P.S. has received investigator fees and/or advisory board member and/or consultancy and/or travel grants from Allergan-Abbvie, Novartis, Elli-Lilly, and Teva. P.L. has received investigator fees and/or advisory board member and/or consultancy and/or travel grants from Allergan-Abbvie and Novartis. D.R. (Dimitrios Rikos) has received investigator fees and/or advisory board member and/or consultancy and/or travel grants from Allergan-Abbvie, Novartis, Pfizer, Elli-Lilly, and Teva. A.A.A. has received investigator fees and/or advisory board member and/or consultancy and/or travel grants from Allergan-Abbvie, Elli-Lilly, Novartis, Teva, Lundbeck, and Pfizer.

Institutional Review Board Statement: The study was conducted in accordance with the Declaration of Helsinki. The study protocol was approved by the Institutional Review Board of "Agios Andreas" Patras General Hospital (91/14-12-2022).

Informed Consent Statement: Informed consent was obtained from all subjects involved in the study.

Data Availability Statement: The data that support the findings of this study are available from the corresponding author upon reasonable request.

Conflicts of Interest: The authors declare no conflict of interest.

References

1. Ashina, M.; Terwindt, G.M.; Al-Karagholi, M.A.-M.; de Boer, I.; Lee, M.J.; Hay, D.L.; Schulte, L.H.; Hadjikhani, N.; Sinclair, A.J.; Ashina, H.; et al. Migraine: Disease characterisation, biomarkers, and precision medicine. *Lancet* 2021, *397*, 1496–1504. [CrossRef] [PubMed]
2. Breslau, N.; Lipton, R.B.; Stewart, W.F.; Schultz, L.R.; Welch, K.M. Comorbidity of migraine and depression: Investigating potential etiology and prognosis. *Neurology* 2003, *60*, 1308–1312. [CrossRef] [PubMed]
3. Buse, D.C.; Silberstein, S.D.; Manack, A.N.; Papapetropoulos, S.; Lipton, R.B. Psychiatric comorbidities of episodic and chronic migraine. *J. Neurol.* 2013, *260*, 1960–1969. [CrossRef] [PubMed]
4. Ashina, S.; Serrano, D.; Lipton, R.B.; Maizels, M.; Manack, A.N.; Turkel, C.C.; Reed, M.L.; Buse, D.C. Depression and risk of transformation of episodic to chronic migraine. *J. Headache Pain* 2012, *13*, 615–624. [CrossRef]
5. Vandervorst, F.; Van Deun, L.; Van Dycke, A.; Paemeleire, K.; Reuter, U.; Schoenen, J.; Versijpt, J. CGRP monoclonal antibodies in migraine: An efficacy and tolerability comparison with standard prophylactic drugs. *J. Headache Pain* 2021, *22*, 128. [CrossRef]
6. Reuter, U.; Ehrlich, M.; Gendolla, A.; Heinze, A.; Klatt, J.; Wen, S.; Hours-Zesiger, P.; Nickisch, J.; Sieder, C.; Hentschke, C.; et al. Erenumab versus topiramate for the prevention of migraine—A randomised, double-blind, active-controlled phase 4 trial. *Cephalalgia* 2022, *42*, 108–118. [CrossRef]
7. Deen, M.; Correnti, E.; Kamm, K.; Kelderman, T.; Papetti, L.; Rubio-Beltrán, E.; Vigneri, S.; Edvinsson, L.; Maassen Van Den Brink, A. Blocking CGRP in migraine patients—A review of pros and cons. *J. Headache Pain* 2017, *18*, 96. [CrossRef]
8. Wang, X.; Chen, Y.; Song, J.; You, C. Efficacy and Safety of Monoclonal Antibody Against Calcitonin Gene-Related Peptide or Its Receptor for Migraine: A Systematic Review and Network Meta-analysis. *Front. Pharmacol.* 2021, *12*, 649143. [CrossRef]
9. Messina, R.; Huessler, E.M.; Puledda, F.; Haghdoost, F.; Lebedeva, E.R.; Diener, H.C. Safety and tolerability of monoclonal antibodies targeting the CGRP pathway and gepants in migraine prevention: A systematic review and network meta-analysis. *Cephalalgia* 2023, *43*, 3331024231152169. [CrossRef]
10. Goadsby, P.J.; Holland, P.R.; Martins-Oliveira, M.; Hoffmann, J.; Schankin, C.; Akerman, S. Pathophysiology of Migraine: A Disorder of Sensory Processing. *Physiol. Rev.* 2017, *97*, 553–622. [CrossRef]
11. Melo-Carrillo, A.; Strassman, A.M.; Nir, R.-R.; Schain, A.J.; Noseda, R.; Stratton, J.; Burstein, R. Fremanezumab-A Humanized Monoclonal Anti-CGRP Antibody-Inhibits Thinly Myelinated (Aδ) But Not Unmyelinated (C) Meningeal Nociceptors. *J. Neurosci.* 2017, *37*, 10587–10596. [CrossRef]
12. Silberstein, S.D.; McAllister, P.; Ning, X.; Faulhaber, N.; Lang, N.; Yeung, P.; Schiemann, J.; Aycardi, E.; Cohen, J.M.; Janka, L.; et al. Safety and Tolerability of Fremanezumab for the Prevention of Migraine: A Pooled Analysis of Phases 2b and 3 Clinical Trials. *Headache* 2019, *59*, 880–890. [CrossRef]
13. Pavelic, A.R.; Wöber, C.; Riederer, F.; Zebenholzer, K. Monoclonal Antibodies against Calcitonin Gene-Related Peptide for Migraine Prophylaxis: A Systematic Review of Real-World Data. *Cells* 2022, *12*, 143. [CrossRef]
14. Lipton, R.B.; Cohen, J.M.; Galic, M.; Seminerio, M.J.; Yeung, P.P.; Aycardi, E.; Bigal, M.E.; Bibeau, K.; Buse, D.C. Effects of fremanezumab in patients with chronic migraine and comorbid depression: Subgroup analysis of the randomized HALO CM study. *Headache* 2021, *61*, 662–672. [CrossRef]
15. Argyriou, A.A.; Dermitzakis, E.V.; Xiromerisiou, G.; Rallis, D.; Soldatos, P.; Litsardopoulos, P.; Vikelis, M. Efficacy and safety of fremanezumab for migraine prophylaxis in patients with at least three previous preventive failures: Prospective, multicenter, real-world data from a Greek registry. *Eur. J. Neurol.* 2023, *30*, 1435–1442. [CrossRef]
16. Argyriou, A.A.; Dermitzakis, E.V.; Xiromerisiou, G.; Rallis, D.; Soldatos, P.; Litsardopoulos, P.; Vikelis, M. Predictors of Response to Fremanezumab in Migraine Patients with at Least Three Previous Preventive Failures: Post Hoc Analysis of a Prospective, Multicenter, Real-World Greek Registry. *J. Clin. Med.* 2023, *12*, 3218. [CrossRef]
17. Teva Pharmaceuticals USA, Inc. Highlights for Prescribing Information. AJOVY TM (Fremanezumab-Vfrm) Injection, for Subcutaneous Use. Initial U.S. 2018. Available online: https://www.accessdata.fda.gov/drugsatfda_docs/label/2018/761089s000lbl.pdf (accessed on 15 May 2023).
18. Argyriou, A.A.; Dermitzakis, E.V.; Xiromerisiou, G.; Vikelis, M. OnabotulinumtoxinA Add-On to Monoclonal Anti-CGRP Antibodies in Treatment-Refractory Chronic Migraine. *Toxins* 2022, *14*, 847. [CrossRef]
19. Vikelis, M.; Dermitzakis, E.V.; Argyriou, A.A.; Rikos, D.; Soldatos, P.; Vlachos, G.S.; Notas, K.; Rudolf, J.; Dardiotis, E.; Karapanayiotides, T.; et al. Consensus article: The opinion of the headache scientific panel of the Hellenic Neurological Society on the use of monoclonal antibodies and small molecules targeting the CGRP pathway in the treatment of migraine and cluster headache in clinical practice. *Arch. Clin. Neurol.* 2023, *31*, 18–28.
20. Arnold, M. Headache Classification Committee of the International Headache Society (IHS) The International Classification of Headache Disorders, 3rd edition. *Cephalalgia* 2018, *38*, 1–211.
21. Stewart, W.F.; Lipton, R.B.; Kolodner, K.; Liberman, J.; Sawyer, J. Reliability of the migraine disability assessment score in a population-based sample of headache sufferers. *Cephalalgia* 1999, *19*, 107–174. [CrossRef]
22. Kosinski, M.; Bayliss, M.S.; Bjorner, J.B.; Ware, J.W., Jr.; Garber, W.H.; Batenhorst, A.; Cady, R.; Dahlöf, C.G.H.; Dowson, A.; Tepper, S. A six-item short-form survey for measuring headache impact: The HIT-6. *Qual. Life Res.* 2003, *12*, 963–974. [CrossRef] [PubMed]
23. Rabin, R.; Charro, F.D. EQ-5D: A measure of health status from the EuroQol Group. *Ann. Med.* 2001, *33*, 337–343. [CrossRef] [PubMed]

24. Zigmond, A.S.; Snaith, R.P. The Hospital Anxiety and Depression Scale. *Acta Psychiatr. Scand.* **1983**, *67*, 361–370. [CrossRef] [PubMed]
25. Hurst, H.; Bolton, J. Assessing the clinical significance of change scores recorded on subjective outcome measures. *J. Manip. Physiol. Ther.* **2004**, *27*, 26–35. [CrossRef] [PubMed]
26. Dworkin, R.H.; Turk, D.C.; Wyrwich, K.W.; Beaton, D.; Cleeland, C.S.; Farrar, J.T.; Haythornthwaite, J.A.; Jensen, M.P.; Kerns, R.D.; Ader, D.N.; et al. Interpreting the clinical importance of treatment outcomes in chronic pain clinical trials: IMMPACT recommendations. *J. Pain* **2008**, *9*, 105–121. [CrossRef]
27. Driessen, M.T.; Cohen, J.M.; Thompson, S.F.; Patterson-Lomba, O.; Seminerio, M.J.; Carr, K.; Totev, T.I.; Sun, R.; Yim, E.; Mu, F.; et al. Real-world effectiveness after initiating fremanezumab treatment in US patients with episodic and chronic migraine or difficult-to-treat migraine. *J. Headache Pain* **2022**, *23*, 56. [CrossRef]
28. Krasenbaum, L.J.; Pedarla, V.L.; Thompson, S.F.; Tangirala, K.; Cohen, J.M.; Driessen, M.T. A real-world study of acute and preventive medication use, adherence, and persistence in patients prescribed fremanezumab in the United States. *J. Headache Pain* **2022**, *23*, 54. [CrossRef]
29. Smitherman, T.A.; Tietjen, G.E.; Schuh, K.; Skljarevski, V.; Lipsius, S.; D'Souza, D.N.; Pearlman, E.M. Efficacy of Galcanezumab for Migraine Prevention in Patients with a Medical History of Anxiety and/or Depression: A Post Hoc Analysis of the Phase 3, Randomized, Double-Blind, Placebo-Controlled REGAIN, and Pooled EVOLVE-1 and EVOLVE-2 Studies. *Headache* **2020**, *60*, 2202–2219. [CrossRef]
30. Yang, Y.; Zhao, H.; Boomsma, D.I.; Ligthart, L.; Belin, A.C.; Smith, G.D.; Esko, T.; Freilinger, T.M.; Hansen, T.F.; Ikram, M.A.; et al. Molecular genetic overlap between migraine and major depressive disorder. *Eur. J. Hum. Genet.* **2018**, *26*, 1202–1216. [CrossRef]
31. Consortium, B.; Anttila, V.; Bulik-Sullivan, B.; Finucane, H.K.; Walters, R.K.; Bras, J.; Duncan, L.; Escott-Price, V.; Falcone, G.J.; Gormley, P.; et al. Analysis of shared heritability in common disorders of the brain. *Science* **2018**, *360*, 8757. [CrossRef]
32. Rossi, C.; Pini, L.A.; Cupini, M.L.; Calabresi, P.; Sarchielli, P. Endocannabinoids in platelets of chronic migraine patients and medication-overuse headache patients: Relation with serotonin levels. *Eur. J. Clin. Pharmacol.* **2008**, *64*, 1–8. [CrossRef]
33. Ren, C.; Liu, J.; Zhou, J.; Liang, H.; Wang, Y.; Sun, Y.; Ma, B.; Yin, Y. Low levels of serum serotonin and amino acids identified in migraine patients. *Biochem. Biophys. Res. Commun.* **2018**, *496*, 267–273. [CrossRef]
34. Gasparini, C.F.; Smith, R.A.; Griffiths, L.R. Genetic and biochemical changes of the serotonergic system in migraine pathobiology. *J. Headache Pain* **2017**, *18*, 20. [CrossRef]
35. Vieira, D.S.; Naffah-Mazacoratti, M.G.; Zukerman, E.; Senne Soares, C.A.; Alonso, E.O.; Faulhaber, M.H.; Cavalheiro, E.A.; Peres, M.F. Cerebrospinal fluid GABA levels in chronic migraine with and without depression. *Brain Res.* **2006**, *1090*, 197–201. [CrossRef]
36. Hamel, E. Serotonin and migraine: Biology and clinical implications. *Cephalalgia* **2007**, *27*, 1293–1300. [CrossRef]
37. Burch, R. Antidepressants for Preventive Treatment of Migraine. *Curr. Treat. Options Neurol.* **2019**, *21*, 18. [CrossRef]
38. Minen, M.T.; Begasse De Dhaem, O.; Kroon Van Diest, A.; Powers, S.; Schwedt, T.J.; Lipton, R.; Silbersweig, D. Migraine and its psychiatric comorbidities. *J. Neurol. Neurosurg. Psychiatry* **2016**, *87*, 741–749. [CrossRef]
39. Altamura, C.; Corbelli, I.; de Tommaso, M.; Di Lorenzo, C.; Di Lorenzo, G.; Di Renzo, A.; Filippi, M.; Jannini, T.B.; Messina, R.; Parisi, P.; et al. Pathophysiological Bases of Comorbidity in Migraine. *Front. Hum. Neurosci.* **2021**, *15*, 640574. [CrossRef]
40. Asif, N.; Patel, A.; Vedantam, D.; Poman, D.S.; Motwani, L. Migraine with Comorbid Depression: Pathogenesis, Clinical Implications, and Treatment. *Cureus* **2022**, *14*, e25998. [CrossRef]
41. Yang, Y.; Zhao, H.; Heath, A.C.; Madden, P.A.; Martin, N.G.; Nyholt, D.R. Familial Aggregation of Migraine and Depression: Insights from a Large Australian Twin Sample. *Twin Res. Hum. Genet.* **2016**, *19*, 312–321. [CrossRef]
42. Sink, K.S.; Walker, D.L.; Yang, Y.; Davis, M. Calcitonin gene-related peptide in the bed nucleus of the stria terminalis produces an anxiety-like pattern of behavior and increases neural activation in anxiety-related structures. *J. Neurosci.* **2011**, *31*, 1802–1810. [CrossRef] [PubMed]
43. Amoozegar, F.; Patten, S.B.; Becker, W.J.; Bulloch, A.G.M.; Fiest, K.M.; Davenport, J.; Carroll, C.R.; Jetté, N. The prevalence of depression and the accuracy of depression screening tools in migraine patients. *Gen. Hosp. Psych.* **2017**, *48*, 25–31. [CrossRef] [PubMed]
44. Yong, N.; Hu, H.; Fan, X.; Li, X.; Ran, L.; Qu, Y.; Wang, Y.; Tan, G.; Chen, L.; Zhou, J. Prevalence and risk factors for depression and anxiety among outpatient migraineurs in mainland China. *J. Headache Pain* **2012**, *13*, 303–310. [CrossRef] [PubMed]
45. Sajobi, T.T.; Amoozegar, F.; Wang, M.; Wiebe, N.; Fiest, K.M.; Patten, S.B.; Jette, N. Global assessment of migraine severity measure: Preliminary evidence of construct validity. *BMC Neurol.* **2019**, *19*, 53. [CrossRef] [PubMed]
46. From clinicaltrials.gov: A Study to Evaluate the Efficacy and Safety of Fremanezumab for Preventive Treatment of Migraine in Patients with Major Depressive Disorder. ClinicalTrials.gov Identifier: NCT04041284. Available online: https://clinicaltrials.gov/ct2/show/NCT04041284 (accessed on 15 May 2023).

Disclaimer/Publisher's Note: The statements, opinions and data contained in all publications are solely those of the individual author(s) and contributor(s) and not of MDPI and/or the editor(s). MDPI and/or the editor(s) disclaim responsibility for any injury to people or property resulting from any ideas, methods, instructions or products referred to in the content.

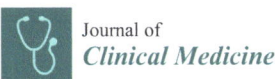

Article

A Novel Virtual-Based Comprehensive Clinical Approach to Headache Care

Thomas Berk [1,2,*], Stephen Silberstein [2] and Peter McAllister [3]

[1] Neura Health, New York, NY 10017, USA
[2] Jefferson Headache Center, Thomas Jefferson University, Philadelphia, PA 19107, USA
[3] New England Institute for Neurology and Headache, Stamford, CT 06905, USA; peter@neinh.com
* Correspondence: tom@neurahealth.co; Tel.: +1-313-887-0960

Abstract: One major innovation, a result of the coronavirus pandemic, has been the proliferation of telemedicine. Telehealth can help solve the access problems that plague headache medicine, allowing patients in areas with no headache expertise to consult and work with a headache specialist. This is a retrospective chart review of patients seen by Neura Health, a comprehensive app-based telehealth headache center. Patients are seen by a specialist and, in addition to any medical recommendations, are given care plans individualized to their condition and recommendations at the end of their clinical appointments. The primary outcome of this study is a decrease in monthly headache days after 90 days; secondary outcomes include disability as determined by MIDAS score, depression determined by PHQ-9, patients' utilization of emergency department or urgent care resources, as well as their global impression of improvement. The deidentified outcomes of consecutive patients of Neura Health were evaluated from March 2022–March 2023. Subjects were excluded if they did not complete all forms, or if they did not receive a clinical or coaching follow-up appointment within 90 days. A total of 186 consecutive patients at Neura Health were identified during the review period. The median decrease in monthly headache days was 55.0% after a 90 day period, headache severity was decreased by 16.7%, global impression of improvement increased by 60.9%, disability decreased by 38.7%, depression decreased by 12.5% and ER/urgent care visits were decreased by 66.1%. A comprehensive, telehealth-based virtual headache-care model significantly decreased migraine frequency, severity and disability, and is able to decrease ER or urgent care visits.

Keywords: headache; migraine; telehealth; virtual care; coaching

1. Introduction

Migraine is a leading cause of disability; headache disorders, according to the World Health Organization, are some of the most common disease conditions worldwide [1]. Headache affects nearly everyone at some point in their lives and migraine, specifically, is estimated to affect over 1 billion people globally [2]. The understanding and treatment of headache disorders has improved significantly over the past few decades, with disease-specific preventive and acute treatments now available.

Although our understanding of headache conditions has improved, and we are now able to treat them on a molecular level, the evaluation of headache disorders remains unchanged for the past 40 years. Most people with headache are not evaluated by a neurologist or headache specialist. They are often misunderstood or misdiagnosed by a primary care provider or emergency care provider. Those without access to specialty care often end up self-medicating with over-the-counter treatments that not only do not prevent the attacks from happening, but often worsen the underlying condition due to medication adaptation and overuse.

Access to specialists is mainly determined by a person's geographic location [3]. It is much more difficult, if not near impossible, for people from rural locations, or even larger cities that do not have a headache specialist, to be seen by someone with expertise in headache conditions. Prior studies have shown significant improvement in the outcomes of patients followed by neurologists or headache specialists versus primary care physicians.

The recent COVID-19 pandemic resulted in the proliferation of virtual medical care. The use of telehealth was estimated to have grown by 15 times from 2019 to 2021. Prior to 2019, telehealth was used primarily as a means of access by patients in remote locations [4]. During the height of the pandemic, many physicians and patients used telehealth for continuity of care.

Some medical subspecialties are more appropriate for virtual care. Psychiatry has flourished in this virtual world, with many psychiatrists not planning to return to in-person visits [5,6]. Within neurology, headache medicine, and the treatment of migraine specifically is well suited for virtual care [7]. The typical age of patients with migraine and other headache conditions is the second to fourth decade, a population that is more technically savvy. This population generally consists of people that are otherwise healthy and generally have normal neurological exam findings. The majority of people with headache conditions do not require interventional therapies such as in-office injections. Telehealth can also solve the access problems that plague headache medicine and other neurological subspecialties, allowing patients in areas without a headache specialist to now have this option.

Telehealth allows a more comprehensive approach to the treatment of headache disorders. In a traditional setting, when a patient sees their doctor intermittently, the focus of the appointment is the diagnosis and medical treatment of their headache disorder. Despite the best intentions of the physician, and due to constraints beyond their control, the appointments often feel rushed, and it is more difficult to comprehensively treat patients, to fully educate them on their condition, including the appropriate non-medical options that are available for them. In a virtual setting, patient appointments are on time more often and patients can more easily be sent additional education material; in addition to their medications, patients are given an app-based, comprehensive curriculum focused on their needs. These can include neck and shoulder exercises, stress management if appropriate, relaxation strategies, and vestibular exercises. Telehealth can also improve access, as rural areas were some of the earliest adopters of telehealth appointments, well before the pandemic [4].

Despite these advantages, telehealth is not an option for all patients. Photophobia is the most common migraine-associated sensitivity, and often screen use can be a triggering activity for people with migraine. People with secondary headache disorders necessarily need further interventions including urgent imaging and a hands-on, in-person evaluation. These can often be accounted for by giving patients instructions on how to make their screens less triggering (dimming the lights, using "nightshift" mode) and by implementing strict guidelines to quickly recognize secondary headache conditions and refer them appropriately for in-person interventions.

Neura Health was founded in 2020 as the first ever comprehensive headache center that is virtual and based on telehealth. Providers are UCNS-certified or fellowship-trained MDs, or physician assistants that have extensive training and work experience at headache centers. Physicians are licensed in most states of the United States; they can offer "educational appointments" to patients located outside of those states and Neura Health providers can work together with the patient's local physicians to provide them their prescriptions and evidenced-based recommendations. Neura's providers follow strict protocols that are based on the American Academy of Neurology and American Headache Society's best practice guidelines.

Few outcome studies exist for telehealth with respect to headache. This retrospective chart review is intended to help determine the effectiveness of a comprehensive approach to headache care, provided via telehealth.

2. Materials and Methods

2.1. Virtual Comprehensive Headache Center

Neura Health is a telehealth-based model of neurological care. Similar to an in-person evaluation, headache patients can make an appointment to see a neurologist or headache specialist that is either licensed in their state or that can work with the patient's local doctors. During their virtual patient encounter, they are given a standardized virtual neurological exam, testing eye movement, facial symmetry, tongue and palate movement, drift, fine finger movement, coordination, upper and lower extremity strength, balance and gait. Medication, laboratory testing and imaging recommendations are also standardized as per the American Headache Society and American Academy of Neurology guidelines and best practices.

All patients are given care plans individualized to their unique needs at the end of their clinical appointments. These include information regarding starting or adjusting medications, and information about any prescribed medications and the underlying headache condition with which they are being diagnosed. Patients are provided with an individualized 90-day educational curriculum focusing on symptom tracking/calendaring via a proprietary headache calendar, biofeedback, physical therapy exercises specific for their specific headache condition (such as migraine, tension type or cervicogenic headache) or diet-based recommendations.

In addition, each patient is assigned a certified health coach that they can meet with on a twice-monthly basis. All Neura Health coaches are NBC-HWC trained and certified, and undergo a headache-specific training process to learn evidence-based, non-medical recommendations for headache conditions. Patients meet with their coaches for 20–30 min via video conference twice monthly, for supportive care, accountability regarding their care plans, and for goal setting based on the patients' specific needs for the next 2 weeks. Care teams are alerted if the patient reports worsening when tracking their headaches, and work with their patients to determine what potential non-medical options may be helpful.

2.2. Clinical Trial

Subject Identification

The deidentified outcomes of consecutive patients of Neura Health were evaluated from March 2022–March 2023. Subjects with all headache disorders were included in this evaluation. An intake questionnaire is given to all patients prior to their first appointment, and patients also receive a weekly check-in questionnaire and a 90-day questionnaire. Subjects also included if they had an undifferentiated headache disorder awaiting a diagnostic test or treatment to determine their headache diagnosis.

Subjects were excluded if they did not complete all forms, or if they did not receive a clinical or coaching follow-up appointment within 90 days. An interim evaluation was performed to determine if any subject's data were 2 standard deviations outside the mean; these subjects were excluded as well.

During their initial questionnaire, patients are asked to self-identify their current baseline frequency of headache days, severity based on a visual analogue scale, as well as the number of emergency department or urgent care visits over the past 90 days. Patients were also asked their global impression of improvement ("How close do you feel to finding relief?"). They are also given a MIDAS and PHQ-9 questionnaire to determine their baseline level of migraine associated disability and depression. Patients are asked weekly if they feel that their symptoms are improving or worsening, how severe and frequent they were on average that past week, and if they went to an emergency room or urgent care center. At 90 days, patients are asked again for their frequency of monthly headache days, average severity, global impression of improvement, MIDAS and PHQ-9.

Patients of all headache conditions and diagnoses were included, including undifferentiated headache conditions that required a confirmatory test or referral to an outside provider. These referrals were expeditiously made to local in-person providers, including ophthalmologists, endocrinologists, orthopedic or neurological spine surgeons or, if urgent, to a local emergency department. Imaging was ordered following the American Headache Society 2019 Neuroimaging Guidelines [8].

2.3. Outcomes Evaluation

The primary outcome for this study was mean decrease in monthly headache days after 90 days. Secondary outcomes were mean decrease in headache-related disability as determined by MIDAS score, mean decrease in headache severity, decrease in depression as determined by PHQ-9 score and decrease in emergency room or urgent care visits also after 90 days. Demographic information was evaluated including age, gender and ethnicity.

2.4. Statistical Evaluation

A two-tailed *t*-test was performed for all variables as noted above. The significance of alpha was determined at $p < 0.01$ with 95% confidence intervals (CI). Data analysis was performed using Big Query v3.14.0. Three predetermined interval statistical reviews were performed to recognize significant outliers, defined as outcomes more than 2 standard deviations outside of the mean.

2.5. Ethics Statement

This study was determined to have a D4-IRB exemption as per the WCG IRB Affairs Department. This exemption is under 45 CFR § 46.104(d)(4), "because the research involves the use of identifiable private information/biospecimens; and information, which may include information about biospecimens, is recorded by the investigator in such a manner that the identity of the human subjects cannot readily by ascertained directly or through identifiers linked to the subjects, the investigator does not contact the subjects, and the investigator will not re-identify subjects."

3. Results

3.1. Study Design and Participants

A total of 186 consecutive Neura Health patients were identified during the review period. The data of 117 subjects were included. Exclusions were primarily due to incomplete forms at intake or after 90 days, or lack of a follow-up appointment within 90 days. Patients with secondary headaches were included after confirmation from an in-person specialist when appropriate.

3.2. Statistical Review

Three interim reviews were performed by a third-party data analyst. These were performed at predetermined intervals—at 50%, 75% and 90% of data collection. The purpose of the interim reviews was to exclude very significant data errors, defined as outliers 2 standard deviations outside of the mean. A total of four subjects were excluded after these analyses (Table 1).

Table 1. Demographics.

Sex (%)	Female (%)	Male (%)	Non-Binary (%)		
	101 (86.3)	15 (12.8)	1 (0.9)		
Race	Caucasian (%)	Black/African American (%)	Asian (%)	Native American (%)	Other (%)
	92 (78.6)	3 (2.6)	9 (7.7)	1 (0.9)	11 (9.4)
Age	0–20 (%)	21–30 (%)	31–40 (%)	41–50 (%)	51–60 (%)	65+ (%)
	4 (3.4)	23 (19.7)	34 (29.1)	25 (21.4)	19 (16.2)	12 (10.3)

3.3. Demographics

An overview of the demographics of this population can be found in Table 1. This study population had 101 females (86.3%, 12.8% male and 0.9% nonbinary individuals), and a median age of 42.0 years (14–93). An amount of 78.6% identified as Caucasian, 2.6% African American, 7.7% Asian, 0/9% Native American and 9.4% other.

3.4. Baseline Headache Data

The mean frequency of this study population was significantly higher than expected (18 monthly headache days). The mean attack severity was 6.5 out of 10, mean MIDAS was 62.0 and PHQ-9 was 8.0. There was an average of 0.5 ER or urgent care visits in the past 90 days, and the global impression of improvement at baseline ("Relief") was 3.0 out of 10.

3.5. Primary and Secondary Outcomes

Mean decrease in monthly headache days was 29.0%, and median decrease was 55.0% after 90 days ($p = 0$, 95%CI), from 18 to 9 days per month (Table 2). Mean severity decreased 15.3%, median severity decreased by 16.7% ($p = 0.01$, 95% CI) and global impression of improvement increased an average of 60.9%; the median improvement was 100% ($p = 0$, 95% CI).

Table 2. Headache frequency, severity, disability, relief and depression.

Frequency (Monthly Headache Days)	Median % Decrease (Range from Baseline)	Mean % Decrease (Range from Baseline)	$p =$
	55.0 (20–9)	29.0 (17.6–12.5)	0.00
Severity	Median % decrease (range from baseline)	Mean % decrease (range from baseline)	$p =$
	16.7 (6–5)	15.3 (6.1–5.2)	0.01
MIDAS	Median % decrease (range from baseline)	Mean % decrease (range from baseline)	$p =$
	38.7 (62–38)	12.8 (89.5–78.1)	0.00
Global Impression of improvement	Median % change (range from baseline)	Mean % decrease (range from baseline)	$p =$
	100 (3–6)	60.9 (3.4–5.5)	0.00
PHQ-9	Median % decrease (range from baseline)	Mean % decrease (range from baseline)	$p =$
	12.5 (8–7)	8.7 (8.4–7.6)	0.01

3.6. Other Secondary Outcomes

Mean PHQ-9 score decreased by 8.7%, the median decrease was 12.5% ($p = 0.01$, 95% CI), disability as measured by MIDAS decreased by an average of 12.8%, and the median's decrease was 38.7% ($p = 0.01$, 95% CI). ER and urgent care visits were decreased by 66.1% ($p = 0$, 95% CI).

4. Discussion

Telehealth is widely used in some neurological subspecialties such as stroke to provide specialty expertise in remote settings. Over the course of the COVID pandemic, telehealth was relied upon out of necessity in many clinical settings where it was not previously used. The American Academy of Neurology has provided a position statement strongly in favor of utilizing and expanding virtual care.

Prior outcomes regarding telehealth have been rare, but positive (See Table 3). During the COVID-19 pandemic, telehealth was in its infancy, and could be optimized further with future innovations. We believe that the comprehensive nature of our care model is part of the future of headache care.

Table 3. Publications on telehealth.

Publication, Author	Year	Title	Outcome
Chiang, Halker Singh et al. [7]	2021	Patient experience of telemedicine for headache care during the COVID-19 pandemic: An American Migraine Foundation survey study	Telemedicine facilitated headache care for many patients during the COVID-19 pandemic, resulting in high patient satisfaction rates, and a desire to continue to use telemedicine for future headache care among those who completed the online survey.
Grinberg, Fenton et al. [9]	2022	Telehealth perceptions and utilization for the delivery of headache care before and during the COVID-19 pandemic: A mixed-methods study	Patients and providers were amenable to utilizing telehealth, yet also experienced technological barriers
Noutsios, Boisvert-Plante et al. [10]	2021	Telemedicine Applications for the Evaluation of Patients with Non-Acute Headache: A Narrative Review	High satisfaction rates have been reported for virtual headache management which were shown to be equal to in-person consults.
Minen, Szperka et al. [11]	2021	Telehealth as a new care delivery model: The headache provider experience	Respondents were comfortable treating patients with migraine via telehealth. They note positive attributes for patients and how access may be improved.

We present the first outcomes data specifically reviewing headache telehealth. This trial included patients with any headache disorder or diagnosis (migraine, tension type headache, as well as SUNCT and intracranial hypotension), all primary and secondary headache conditions. "Red flags" of headache were screened for during the virtual appointment, and any concerning finding was referred for appropriate in-person intervention or evaluation. The decision to recommend imaging was based on the American Headache Society Imaging Guidelines, in order to not over utilize imaging modalities.

This study population had a very high baseline monthly headache frequency and severity, similar to a tertiary headache center. Despite the severity of this population, there was a significant improvement in all outcomes measured. We feel that, in particular, a high severity population can benefit more from a virtual platform due to the comprehensive nature of the treatment, and the ability to avoid triggering commutes to in-person doctor's appointments which are often triggering with bright lights, loud noises and smells.

This comprehensive approach to headache disorders has revealed statistically significant and beneficial outcomes with a decreases in monthly headache days, migraine-related disability, depression, and ER/urgent care visitation. Statistically significant, but less robust, was the decrease in overall headache intensity. We believe that this is most likely due to our inclusion of a number of refractory chronic headache disorders such as chronic migraine and intracranial hypotension. The focus when treating these chronic disorders is primarily on decreasing monthly headache days, more than improvement in the severity of each attack.

We believe that there are many significant advantages to a virtual approach to headache disorders. Many patients started seeing their medical professionals virtually over this period of time, and they appreciated avoiding the time and cost of commuting to the doctor's office. Recent studies have highlighted the fact that most patients prefer many aspects of telehealth visits over in-person visits.

In addition to convenience, we have been able to develop a more comprehensive approach to headache care via telehealth. Patients receive a comprehensive educational curriculum, specific care plans related to their own unique issues, and individualized coaching. Although it is possible to develop similar protocols in a traditional office setting, telehealth has allowed this to be performed in a very efficient, comprehensive, and convenient process.

There are limiting factors to telehealth for headache conditions. In-person procedures and infusions must be referred to a local physician or center. Licensing across state lines can be expensive or time consuming, and state and federal regulations regarding virtual medical care are frequently changing. Providers may be concerned that although reimbursements of virtual care are currently the same as in-person appointments, this may change in the future.

Not all patients are appropriate for telehealth as well, as noted above. Patients with severe photophobia may not be able to tolerate screens at all, even with adjustments to the brightness or blue-light filtering. Patients with concern for secondary headache conditions will still need to be evaluated in person, and with appropriate referrals and imaging. Depending on the secondary etiology, they may not be appropriate to be followed long term virtually and may need an in-person specialist.

Technology is innovating much of what we do on a new daily basis. As we look to the future of medical care, we must consider ways to excel and give our patients the best likelihood for better outcomes. Leveraging telehealth's opportunities for comprehensive and individualized care is one important step in this direction.

Author Contributions: Conceptualization, T.B.; methodology, T.B. and P.M.; software, T.B.; validation, T.B.; formal analysis, T.B.; investigation, S.S.; resources, S.S.; data curation, T.B.; writing—original draft preparation, T.B.; writing—review and editing, P.M. and S.S. All authors have read and agreed to the published version of the manuscript.

Funding: This research received no external funding.

Institutional Review Board Statement: This study was determined to have a D4-IRB exemption as per the WCG IRB Affairs Department. This exemption is under 45 CFR § 46.104(d)(4), because the research involves the use of identifiable private information/biospecimens; and information, which may include information about biospecimens, is recorded by the investigator in such a manner that the identity of the human subjects cannot readily by ascertained directly or through identifiers linked to the subjects, the investigator does not contact the subjects, and the investigator will not re-identify subjects.

Informed Consent Statement: Informed consent was obtained from all subjects involved in the study.

Data Availability Statement: The data presented in this study are available on request from the corresponding author. The data are not publicly available due to HIPPA and the potential of patient identification.

Acknowledgments: The authors thank Elizabeth Burstein and Sameer Madan, the co-founders of Neura Health. We also acknowledge the hard work and dedication of the physicians, coaches and physician assistants at Neura Health.

Conflicts of Interest: T.B. is an employee of Neura Health, P.M. is an advisor and has received equity. S.S. has no conflict of interest.

References

1. GBD Chronic Kidney Disease Collaboration. Global, regional, and national burden of chronic kidney disease, 1990–2017: A systematic analysis for the Global Burden of Disease Study 2017. *Lancet* **2020**, *395*, 709–733. [CrossRef] [PubMed]
2. Ashina, M.; Katsarava, Z.; Do, T.P.; Buse, D.C.; Pozo-Rosich, P.; Özge, A.; Krymchantowski, A.V.; Lebedeva, E.R.; Ravishankar, K.; Yu, S.; et al. Migraine: Epidemiology and systems of care. *Lancet* **2021**, *397*, 1485–1495. [CrossRef] [PubMed]
3. Vgontzas, A.; Loder, E. Addressing inequities in headache care by embedding services in a community health center in Boston, MA. *Headache* **2022**, *62*, 1416–1418. [CrossRef] [PubMed]
4. Shaver, J. The State of Telehealth Before and After the COVID-19 Pandemic. *Prim. Care* **2022**, *49*, 517–530. [CrossRef] [PubMed]
5. de Oliveira, P.B.F.; Dornelles, T.M.; Gosmann, N.P.; Camozzato, A. Efficacy of telemedicine interventions for depression and anxiety in older people: A systematic review and meta-analysis. *Int. J. Geriatr. Psychiatry* **2023**, *38*, e5920. [CrossRef] [PubMed]

6. Kamma, H.K.; Alabbas, M.; Elashahab, M.; Abid, N.; Manaye, S.; Cheran, K.; Murthy, C.; Bornemann, E.A.; Franchini, A.P.A. The Efficacy of Telepsychiatry in Addiction Patients: A Systematic Review. *Cureus* **2023**, *15*, e38133. [CrossRef] [PubMed]
7. Chiang, C.; Singh, R.H.; Lalvani, N.; Stein, K.S.; Lorenz, D.H.; Lay, C.; Dodick, D.W.; Newman, L.C. Patient experience of telemedicine for headache care during the COVID-19 pandemic: An American Migraine Foundation survey study. *Headache* **2021**, *61*, 734–739. [CrossRef] [PubMed]
8. Evans, R.W.; Burch, R.C.; Frishberg, B.M.; Marmura, M.J.; Mechtler, L.L.; Silberstein, S.D.; Turner, D.P. Neuroimaging for Migraine: The American Headache Society Systematic Review and Evidence-Based Guideline. *Headache* **2020**, *60*, 318–336. [CrossRef] [PubMed]
9. Grinberg, A.S.; Fenton, B.T.; Wang, K.; Lindsey, H.; Goldman, R.E.; Baird, S.; Riley, S.; Burrone, L.; Seng, E.K.; Damush, T.M.; et al. Telehealth perceptions and utilization for the delivery of headache care before and during the COVID-19 pandemic: A mixed-methods study. *Headache* **2022**, *62*, 613–623. [CrossRef] [PubMed]
10. Noutsios, C.D.; Boisvert-Plante, V.; Perez, J.; Hudon, J.; Ingelmo, P. Telemedicine Applications for the Evaluation of Patients with Non-Acute Headache: A Narrative Review. *J. Pain Res.* **2021**, *14*, 1533–1542. [CrossRef] [PubMed]
11. Minen, M.T.; Szperka, C.L.; Kaplan, K.; Ehrlich, A.; Riggins, N.; Rizzoli, P.; Strauss, L.D. Telehealth as a new care delivery model: The headache provider experience. *Headache* **2021**, *61*, 1123–1131. [CrossRef] [PubMed]

Disclaimer/Publisher's Note: The statements, opinions and data contained in all publications are solely those of the individual author(s) and contributor(s) and not of MDPI and/or the editor(s). MDPI and/or the editor(s) disclaim responsibility for any injury to people or property resulting from any ideas, methods, instructions or products referred to in the content.

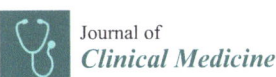

Review

The Dawn and Advancement of the Knowledge of the Genetics of Migraine

Nader G. Zalaquett [1,†], Elio Salameh [1,†], Jonathan M. Kim [2,†], Elham Ghanbarian [3], Karen Tawk [2,*] and Mehdi Abouzari [2,*]

1. Faculty of Medicine, American University of Beirut, Beirut 1107, Lebanon
2. Department of Otolaryngology-Head and Neck Surgery, University of California, Irvine, CA 92697, USA
3. Department of Neurology, University of California, Irvine, CA 92617, USA
* Correspondence: ktawk@hs.uci.edu (K.T.); mabouzar@hs.uci.edu (M.A.)
† These authors contributed equally to this manuscript.

Abstract: Background: Migraine is a prevalent episodic brain disorder known for recurrent attacks of unilateral headaches, accompanied by complaints of photophobia, phonophobia, nausea, and vomiting. Two main categories of migraine are migraine with aura (MA) and migraine without aura (MO). **Main body:** Early twin and population studies have shown a genetic basis for these disorders, and efforts have been invested since to discern the genes involved. Many techniques, including candidate-gene association studies, loci linkage studies, genome-wide association, and transcription studies, have been used for this goal. As a result, several genes were pinned with concurrent and conflicting data among studies. It is important to understand the evolution of techniques and their findings. **Conclusions:** This review provides a chronological understanding of the different techniques used from the dawn of migraine genetic investigations and the genes linked with the migraine subtypes.

Keywords: migraine; migraine with aura (MA); migraine without aura (MO); familial hemiplegic migraine (FHM); genetics

1. Introduction

Migraine is a common episodic brain disorder known for its attacks of severe unilateral headaches, accompanied by photophobia, phonophobia, nausea, and vomiting [1–3]. According to the Global Burden of Disease Study in 2020, migraine remains second among the etiologies of disability [4,5], affecting 18% of women and 6% of men. Two prevalent types of migraine are migraine with aura (MA) and migraine without aura (MO). MA is a severe headache preceded by transient neurologic symptoms such as visual, sensory, and speech disturbances, which are not found in MO [6]. In addition, in the latest International Headache Society (IHS) criteria, MA includes motor and brainstem symptoms [1] (Table 1). The possible underlying mechanism of the aura is a brief wave of nervous system cell depolarization, propagating to the zones in the occipital lobe (cortical spreading depolarization), including the visual cortex, leading to the suppression of brain activity [7]. The exact relationship between cortical spreading depression (CSD) and headache is unknown, but there is evidence that CSD activates trigeminal nociceptors in rats [8,9].

Clinically, MA and MO are two different diagnosable entities, with the latter being more prevalent [10]. The international classification of headache disorder (ICHD-3) criteria for the diagnosis of the mentioned types of migraine are shown in Table 1 [11]. However, there is a historical unsettled debate on whether MO and MA are different disease entities or different manifestations of the same disease. This debate, while not directly related to the genetic basis of migraine, is an important aspect of the overall understanding of the condition and its subtypes.

Table 1. a. ICHD-3 criteria for migraine with aura diagnosis [11]. b. ICHD-3 criteria for migraine without aura diagnosis.

a
A. At least 2 attacks fulfilling criteria B and C

B. One or more of the following fully reversible aura symptoms:
  1. Visual
  2. Sensory
  3. Speech and/or language
  4. Motor
  5. Brainstem
  6. Retinal

C. At least 2 of the following 4 characteristics:
  1. At least 1 aura symptom spreads gradually over greater than or equal to 5 m, and/or more symptoms occur in succession
  2. Each individual aura symptom lasts 5–60 m
  3. At least 1 aura symptom is unilateral
  4. The aura is accompanied, or followed within 60 m, by a headache

D. Not better accounted for by another ICHD-3 diagnosis, and transient ischemic attack has been excluded
b
A. At least 5 attacks fulfilling criteria B–D
B. Headache attacks lasting 4–72 h (when untreated or unsuccessfully treated)
C. Headache has at 2 two of the following 4 characteristics:
1. Unilateral location
2. Pulsating quality
3. Moderate or severe pain intensity
4. Aggravation by or causing avoidance of routine physical activity (e.g., walking or climbing stairs)
D. During headache at least one of the following occurs:
1. Nausea and/or vomiting
2. Photophobia and phonophobia
E. Not better accounted for by another ICHD-3 diagnosis

Note 1: When, for example, 3 symptoms occur during an aura, the acceptable maximal duration is 3 × 60 m. Motor symptoms may last up to 72 h. Aphasia is always regarded as a unilateral symptom, dysarthria may or may not be. Note 2: One or a few migraine attacks may be difficult to distinguish from symptomatic migraine-like attacks. Furthermore, the nature of a single or a few attacks may be difficult to understand. Therefore, at least five attacks are required. Individuals who otherwise meet the criteria for 1.1 Migraine without aura but have had fewer than five attacks should be coded 1.5.1 Probable migraine without aura. When the patient falls asleep during a migraine attack and wakes up without it, the duration of the attack is reckoned until the time of awakening. In children and adolescents (aged under 18 years), attacks may last 2–72 h (the evidence for untreated durations of less than two hours in children has not been substantiated).

Hemiplegic migraine, a debilitating chronic disorder diagnosed as familial (FHM) or sporadic (SHM), is a rare condition that comprises an aura and migraine stage. Affected individuals usually experience reversible neurological symptoms [12], such as hemiplegia or motor impairment, in the aura phase before the onset of migraine headaches [1,11]. The familial variant, an inherited autosomal dominant channelopathy [13], affects an individual's first- or second-degree relatives [14], and can be divided into three unique types as follows [15]:

(1) FHM1 defined by mutations in the CACNA1A gene in chromosome 19,
(2) FHM2 with a mutant ATP1A2 gene in chromosome 1,
(3) FHM3 with SCN1A mutations in chromosome 2.

Although the genes implicated in the familial form are quite well understood [16,17], their role in conjunction with other unknown genes in the sporadic form is relatively obscure [18]. Sporadic hemiplegic migraine is akin to the familial version in that both share clinical commonalities and, in some cases, genetic causes [19]. To illustrate, a 57-year-old women, who displayed an array of symptoms, such as hemiparesis, had a genetic mutation (T1174s) in the sodium voltage-gated channel gene (SCN1A), which led to a sporadic hemiplegic migraine diagnosis; the aforementioned gene is also implicated in familial hemiplegic migraine, which suggests a genetic overlap between the two hemiplegic migraine variants [20]. Although many studies have found analogies between the two variants [21,22], the full extent of the genetic basis for the sporadic version remains contentious [23].

In this article, we aim to review the literature on the genetics of migraine. The goal of this review is to provide a chronological perspective on the advancements in the genetics of MO and MA since their first investigation. In addition, we aim to discuss the current knowledge of familial hemiplegic migraine.

2. Migraine without Aura and Migraine with Aura

The first population study on MO/MA genetics was published by Rasmussen et al. in 1992 [24], and the first twin study was published in 1998 by Ziegler et al. [25]. In 1995, the first candidate-gene association study (CGAS) was conducted by Frosst et al. [26]; however, the bulk of CGAS migraine research was published after the year 2004 [27–36]. Then, linkage studies, latent class analyses, and trait component analyses were adapted [37–39]. Finally, genome-wide association studies (GWAS), RNA sequencing, and exome/genome sequencing studies were applied to migraine genetics in 2010, 2016, and 2019 by Anttila et al. [40], Perry et al. [41], and Williams et al. [42], respectively. In this section, we will delve deeper into the findings of every research technique in migraine genetics. Figure 1 displays the chronology of MO/MA genetics research.

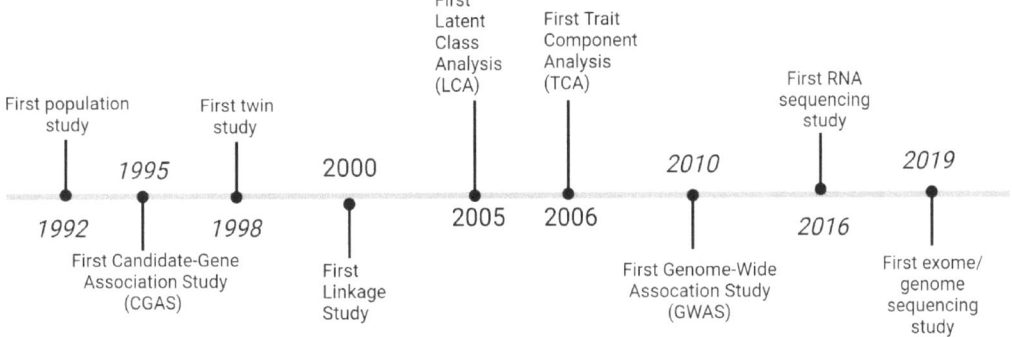

Figure 1. Chronology of techniques used to investigate migraine genetics.

2.1. Genetic Load of MO and MA

Migraine has long been observed to cluster in families, with several patients having their first-degree relatives affected by the condition [43]. Starting in the 1990s, migraine and its genetic mechanism has been demonstrated by twin, family, and population studies [25,43–48]. Population-based studies have shown an increase in familial migraine risk [24,44–46,49]. Indeed, the risk of migraine was 50% higher in relatives of migraine probands [46]. Russel et al. showed that first-degree relatives of patients with MO had approximately a two-fold increased risk for MO, and 1.4 times the risk of having MA. In contrast, they showed that first-degree relatives of patients with MA had a four-fold increase in MA risk, but no increased risk for MO [44]. In addition, another study found a three-fold increase in the risk of MO and a two-fold increase in the risk of MA among first-degree relatives [24,43,49]. Additionally, twin studies provided a great insight into the heritability of migraine. For instance, Gervil et al. and Ulrich et al. analyzed Danish twin populations for the inheritance of MO and MA, respectively [48,50]. The results showed a higher pairwise concordance rate in monozygotic twins (MZ) when compared to dizygotic twins (DZ) (MA $p < 0.001$ and

MO $p < 0.05$) (Table 2) [47,48,50–52]. In addition, pro-band-wise concordance was shown to be higher in MZ when compared to DZ in both MO and MA, as well as in different genders. Furthermore, a study of 30,000 twin pairs showed that genetic factors contribute equally to migraine phenotype as compared to the environment [53]. Finally, a recent study published in 2015 showed a heritability rate for migraine of 42% [54]. All of these published data lead to the conclusion that both MO and MA are a combination of genetics and environmental factors (e.g., stress and bright light) [54,55]. In addition, heritability was seen to be higher in migraine with aura than migraine without aura, leading to a higher genetic susceptibility [56–58].

Table 2. Pairwise concordance rate and proband-wise concordance rate in monozygotic (MZ) and dizygotic (DZ) twins, reported by [47,48,50–52]. (Inspired from Russel et al., 2001).

	Men		Women		Overall	
	MZ	DZ	MZ	DZ	MZ	DZ
Migraine with aura						
Pairwise concordance rate	36%	17%	32%	8%	34%	12%
Proband-wise concordance rate	53%	29%	48%	15%	50%	21%
Migraine without aura						
Pairwise concordance rate	17%	8%	33%	23%	28%	18%
Proband-wise concordance rate	29%	15%	50%	37%	43%	31%

Initially, due to the assumption that a migraine trait is a simple Mendelian transmission, several studies have been conducted, but have failed to clearly discern the mode of inheritance [59–61]. For instance, a study suggested a "sex-limited" inheritance of MO [62]. Another study suggested an autosomal recessive inheritance for MO and MA [60]. Several transmission patterns were hypothesized, but it is widely accepted nowadays that migraine is a genetic multifactorial trait [43,45,63]. Several genes have been correlated to MO and/or MA, which will be discussed below.

2.2. Are MO and MA Different Diseases?

Some clinicians might argue that MA and MO are different manifestations of the same disease [64,65]. Indeed, headache symptoms are virtually identical and might co-occur in the same patient [66], and the type of migraine can change over the years (aura attacks may develop in the elderly) [67]. The same prophylactic and treatment drugs are also effective in both [66]. However, each MO and MA has its own diagnostic criteria in the ICHD-3 [11], and genetic studies have shown different genetic loads for both [68,69].

Some studies have shown a common genetic basis for MA and MO. The international Brainstorm consortium, which compared genetic information between 265,218 patients and 784,643 controls, showed a significant genetic correlation between MO and MA [70]. In addition, the analysis of 23,000 single nucleotide polymorphisms (SNPs) showed that the majority of those analyzed were standard in MO and MA patients [71]; recently, Zhao et al. showed similar results by taking into account all available genetic information [72]. Conversely, several studies showed different genetic components for MO and MA [40,73]. Recently, a study analyzed the polygenic risk score of 21 migraine-associated SNPs and showed their association with MO only. However, many argue that research techniques such as genome-wide association studies (GWAS) particularly identify MO genes, as GWAS detects only top potential SNPs [2,3]. This study involved 152 MA patients compared to the 295 MO cases, which might lead to diminished statistical power when detecting MA genes [2]. In conclusion, with the available evidence, MO and MA are more alike than different; however, further studies are needed to discover the causal genes.

3. Various Techniques Unveiling the Genetic Basis of MO and MA

Several techniques have been used to characterize the genetic basis of MO and MA, starting with the population studies described above. The main methods used to reach this goal were as follows:

(1) candidate-gene association studies (CGAS),
(2) linkage studies,
(3) genome-wide association studies (GWAS),
(4) exome/genome sequencing,
(5) RNA and transcriptome sequencing.

3.1. Candidate-Gene Association Studies (CGAS)

For several years, the genetic basis of migraine was analyzed via focusing on hypothesized candidate genes from hypothesized migraine pathophysiological pathways. For instance, migraine has been linked to neurological, vascular, hormonal, and inflammatory pathways [74]. Using CGAS, approximately 100 genes were correlated with migraine [6].

Homocysteine is an excitatory amino acid that plays a role in the pathophysiology of cerebrovascular diseases [75]. Knowing that migraine has a cerebrovascular basis [27], researchers hypothesized that the genes responsible for homocysteine metabolism might be involved in the etiology of migraine. For example, the methylenetetrahydrofolate reductase gene (MTHFR), which is involved in the metabolism of folate, catalyzes the formation of 5-methylenetetrahydrofolate from 5,10-methylenetetrahydrofolate. The latter is the active form of folate and donates a carbon molecule for homocysteine for it to be converted into methionine [76]. A mutation in MTHFR was hypothesized to cause hyperhomocysteinemia and, consequently, migraine. Indeed, Frosst et al. reported an association between the homozygous C667T mutation of MTHFR and hyperhomocysteinemia [26]. Most studies identified the T-allele of the MTHFR C677T polymorphism to correlate with migraine, specifically MA (but no MO) [27–36]. Scher et al. studied 187 MA and 226 MO patients, in addition to 1212 control non-migraineurs. The group showed that the T/T MTHFR genotype was associated with increased odds of MA when compared to controls (odds ratio [OR], 2.05; 95% confidence interval; $p < 0.006$) [32]. Additionally, Lea et al. studied 652 Caucasian migraineurs and showed that the T/T genotype confers an increased risk for MA (OR: 2.0–2.5), but no increased risk for MO ($p > 0.05$) [29]. Conversely, a study by Todt et al. showed no association between the C667T genotype and MA (OR: 0.61–1.25 and $p = 0.45$) [77]. A possible explanation for their results was that their study's sample sizes was composed of migraineurs with severe symptoms, and, thus, the MTHFR C667T allele could be found only in patients with mild to moderate MA [77]. Also, the International Headache Genetics Consortium (IGHC) data showed no clear evidence of MTHFR correlation in the 5175 migraineurs studied using genome-wide association studies (GWAS) [78].

The dopamine system has been hypothesized to be involved in the pathophysiology of migraine [79]. Studies have shown that D1 and D2 dopamine receptors exist in mice's and rats' trigeminal ganglion and trigeminal nucleus [80–82]. Additionally, studies have shown that administering apomorphine or piribedil (dopamine agonists) increases the cerebral blood flow [83,84]. Other animal studies have shown vasodilation in response to low dopamine doses and vasoconstriction with high doses [85]. As a result, researchers investigated the correlation between the genes involved in the dopaminergic pathway and migraine. The dopamine system is a series of steps, starting from phenylalanine and ending with norepinephrine and epinephrine [79]. Within these steps, dopamine is converted to norepinephrine by dopamine-β-hydroxylase (DBH), and norepinephrine is converted to epinephrine by catechol-O-methyltransferase (COMT) [79]. Finally, upon the release of dopamine in the synaptic cleft, a reuptake mechanism is mediated by presynaptic transporters called dopamine transporters (DAT1 and DAT2) [79]. As such, a mutation in any of the above genes would increase dopamine, and scientists hypothesized a potential increased migraine susceptibility. Two case–control studies have found an increased frequency of migraine in individuals with a homozygous COMT c.472 A > G (Val158Met) when compared to those with the Val/Val genotype [86,87]. However, Hagen et al. showed no association between the Val158Met polymorphism and migraine [88]. In addition, a study investigated the correlation of two SNPs, one within the promoter (−1021C→T) and another (+1603C→T) in exon 11 of the DBH gene in two different cohorts [89]. Results showed an association between the allelic and genotypic frequency distribution of DBH SNPs and migraine in both investigated cohorts [89].

Other genes of the serotonergic system, GABA-A receptor system, insulin receptors, estrogen receptors, LDL receptors, and ion transporters correlated with migraine due to their potential role in its pathophysiology and positive study results [66]. However, similarly to the case of MTHFR and COMT, most of the associations were not replicated and were subsequently disproven. For example, the study of 841 MA patients and 884 controls for thousands of genetic markers in 155 ion transport genes by Nyholt et al. was positive initially, but replication in an independent data set was negative [90]. In addition, 21 genes were associated with MA in another study, but the results could not be replicated in a larger data set [2,78]. Two other genes worth mentioning are the insulin receptor gene (INSR, chromosome 19p13) and the LDL receptor gene (19p13.2). These genes were associated with migraine, but were later disproven. The INSR gene was disproven in a sequencing study, and the LDL receptor gene was disproven because it could not be replicated in another study [91–94]. These disappointing results are due to small sample sizes (less than a few hundred cases), a lack of matching the samples for gender, age, and background, and diagnosis issues [2]. The lack of replication of most CGAS studies raises suspicion that other studies may be false positives; thus, other techniques were used to study the genetics of migraine.

3.2. Loci Linkage Studies

3.2.1. Traditional Linkage Studies

Historically, linkage studies have contributed valuable inputs to the genetics of migraine by pinpointing chromosomal loci in families with migraine [66]. Initially, genotyping was achieved using microsatellite markers or genome-wide scans. For example, Russo et al. analyzed the genetics of 10 Italian families with MA and linked the loci 15q11-q13 with their MA diagnosis using regional microsatellite markers [95]. This locus represents the genomic region of three GABA-A receptor genes. Additionally, a study of a migraine family of 106 individuals from northern Sweden linked the 6p12.2-p21 locus with MO and MA through the use of genome-wide scanning [96]. Replication success for these linkage studies has been scarce, except for a few loci [66]. Wessman et al. and Bjornsson et al. pinned the 4q locus in studies involving Finnish and Icelandic families, respectively [97,98]. The Finnish study revealed locus 4q24 and the Icelandic study revealed locus 4q21 (Table 3). However, many unanswered questions remain concerning these loci; it is unclear whether they contain genes for MO, MA, or both. For these reasons, the validity of the traditional linkage studies results is questionable [66]. Other concerns include a high migraine prevalence and the subjective diagnosis of migraine, which can lead to difficulty in obtaining accurate pedigrees that can link migraine genes.

As a result, alternative linkage studies were used to eliminate this controversy, and two prominent alternatives were the latent class analysis (LCA) and trait component analysis (TCA). Using these methods, researchers can identify loci that could explain an underlying pathophysiological mechanism of a specific symptom [66].

Table 3. Summary of traditional linkage studies results (following the International Headache Classification (IHS) classification guidelines).

Articles	Country	Migraine Type	Genotyping Method	Chromosomal Locus
Nyholt et al., 2000 [37]	Australia	MA/MO	Regional microsatellite markers	Xq25-q28
Jones et al., 2001 [99]	USA	MA	Regional microsatellite markers	19p13
Carlsson et al., 2002 [96]	Sweden	MA/MO	Genome-wide scan	6p12.2-p21
Lea et al., 2002 [100]	Australia	MA/MO	Regional microsatellite markers	1q31
Wessman et al., 2002 [97]	Finland	MA	Genome-wide scan	4q24
Björnsson et al., 2003 [98]	Iceland	MO	Genome-wide scan	4q21
Cader, Noble-Topham et al., 2003 [101]	England	MA	Genome-wide scan	11q24
Soragna et al., 2003 [102]	Italy	MO	Genome-wide scan	14q21.2-q22.3
Russo et al., 2005 [95]	Italy	MA	Regional microsatellite markers	15q11-q13
Anttila et al., 2008 [103]	Australia and Finland	MA	Genome-wide scan	10q22-q23

3.2.2. Latent Class Analysis (LCA)

Latent class analysis was introduced to eliminate the dichotomy of migraine diagnosis. This method focuses on multiple factors of migraine, including symptom severity, leading to a spectrum of clinical presentations. For example, Nyholt et al. [38] (frontrunners of LCA) and Ligthart et al. [104] clustered their patients based on migraine severity and associated symptoms. For instance, Nyholt et al. included pulsation in their classification, and classified their sample into four categories as follows: (1) asymptomatic individuals (CL0), (2) patients with a mild form of recurrent non-migrainous headaches (CL1), (3) patients with a moderately severe form of migraine, often without visual aura (CL2), and (4) patients with a severe form of migraine, often with aura (CL3) [38,64]. As expected, more individuals were labeled using the LCA approach, and none that were diagnosed using the IHS classification were missed [66]. Both of these studies pinned the 5q21 locus. The study by Ligthart et al. also reports the 10q22-q23 locus, in addition to another LCA study on the Australian and Finnish population [103]. This locus was reported using traditional linkage studies and TCA studies (Table 3).

3.2.3. Trait Component Analysis (TCA)

As part of the effort to eliminate the diagnostic bias, researchers adopted the TCA method (starting with Palotie et al.) [103]. Similarly, TCA eliminates the dichotomous diagnostic approach of the IHS and uses the questionnaire information more optimally [103]. More specifically, researchers focus on specific trait components, or, in other words, individual clinical symptoms of migraine, and link chromosomal loci to this phenotypic group [39]. This could eliminate clinical heterogeneity and diagnostic issues. Loci 4q24, 17p13, and 10q22-q23 were linked to different migraine phenotypes using the TCA method (Table 4). Interestingly, 4q24 and 10q22-q23 were reported in Finnish and Australian linkage studies, respectively, using the IHS MA classification [97,103]. The latter mutation is the most significant, as it was replicated in Australian and Dutch studies [104]. The remaining gap unfilled by these new phenotyping methods is the identification of gene variants from the loci, which would give insight into the pathophysiology of specific symptoms and migraine in general.

Table 4. Summary of linkage studies performed with latent class analysis (LCA) and trait component analysis (TCA).

	Article	Country	Phenotypic Classification	Chromosome Locus
Latent Class Analysis				
	Nyholt et al., 2005/ Anttila et al., 2006 [38,39]	Australia	Pulsation	5q21
	Anttila et al., 2006/ Anttila et al., 2008 [39,103]	Australia and Finland	Migrainous headache	10q22-q23
	Anttila et al., 2008/ Ligthart et al., 2008 [103,104]	Netherlands	Migrainous headache	10q22-q23
Trait Component Analysis				
	Nyholt et al., 2005/ Anttila et al., 2006 [38,39]	Finland	Age at onset, photophobia, phonophobia, pain intensity, laterality, pulsation	4q24
	Anttila et al., 2006/ Anttila et al., 2008 [39,103]	Finland	Pulsation	17p13
	Anttila et al., 2008/ Ligthart et al., 2008 [103,104]	Australia and Finland	Laterality, pain intensity, phonophobia, photophobia, pulsation, nausea/vomiting	10q22-q23

3.3. Genome-Wide Association Studies

In the last decade, genome-wide association studies (GWAS) contributed significantly to our knowledge of the genetic basis of migraine. Unlike the other techniques, GWAS requires no prior hypothesis about the role of a DNA variant [105]. Instead, hundreds of thousands to millions of SNPs that are roughly equally dispersed in the genome are analyzed for association with a phenotype, and that is by comparing the results to the controls. The association is considered significant if the p-value is $<5 \times 10^{-8}$, according to the GWAS catalog [106]. This method has been effective in gene associations where other studies did not show results [105].

Ten migraine GWAS studies were conducted in the last decade, which were listed with their findings in Table 5 [40,63,73,74,107–112]. The first study was conducted by Anttila et al. in 2010 [40], and it consisted of 2748 patients with MA and 10,747 matched controls obtained from Finland, Germany, and the Netherlands. A single SNP reached genome-wide significance, which was the rs835740 on chromosome 8q22.1 ($p = 5.38 \times 10^{-9}$, OR = 1.23). This finding was replicated in a meta-analysis showing $p = 1.69 \times 10^{-11}$. This SNP is located between two genes implicated in glutamate homeostasis, which are MTDH (astrocyte elevated gene 1, AEG-1) and PGCP (plasma glutamate carboxypeptidase gene). MTDH has been shown to downregulate SLC1A2 (also known as GLT-1 and EAAT2) in cultured astrocytes; the latter gene encodes for the major glutamate transporters in the brain [113,114]. As such, a decrease in the activity of MTDH and/or PGCP (which metabolizes glutamate) will increase glutamate in the synaptic clefts. This was a plausible hypothesis for researchers as this neurotransmitter has been linked to the pathophysiology of migraine [40]. It is important to note that the relationship between MTDH and migraine remains controversial, as the correlation did not reach significance in subsequent studies [63,107]. Additionally, Gupta et al. [109] showed that the variant rs934937 on chromosome 6p24 increases the risk for migraine. This locus encodes for the PHACTR1 gene, which renders carriers susceptible to other vascular diseases, including coronary artery disease, cervical artery dissection, and hypertension. This gene was also suggested by Freilinger et al. [73] to correlate with MO. This gene was thought to affect the vascular system, and further studies have been completed to characterize its pathophysiological mechanism (check the fine mapping section below) [115].

Table 5. Summary of genome-wide association study (GWAS) results.

Article	Phenotype	Genes	Pathway
Anttila et al., 2010 [40]	MA	MTDH	Glutamate transport
		PGCP	Glutamate metabolism
Chasman et al., 2011 [108]	Migraine	TRPM8	Pain related
		LRP1	Neurotransmission
		PRDM16	Tissue structure and function [116]
Freilinger et al., 2012 [73]	MO	MEF2D	Neurotransmission
		ASTN2	TGF-beta signaling
		TGFBR2	TGF-beta signaling
		PHACTR1	Vascular endothelial function
Anttila et al., 2013 [107]	MA/MO	AJAP1	Metalloproteinase → tumor invasion
		TSPAN2	Metalloproteinase → tumor invasion
		FHL5	cAMP regulation
	MO	MMP6	Neurotransmission
		C7ORF10	Glutaric acid excretion
Gormley et al., 2016 [63]	MA/MO	SLC24A3	
		ITPK1	Ion homeostasis
		GJA1	
Gupta et al., 2016 [109] (phenome-wide AS)	Migraine	PHACTR1	Vascular endothelial function
Gerring et al., 2018 [111]	Migraine	NFKBIZ	
		TNFSF10	
		TNFAIP3	Immune system and inflammation
		CXCR4	
		ABCB1	
		NFIL3	
Guo et al., 2020 [109] (GWAS + transcriptome wide AS)	Migraine	ITGB5	
		SMG6	Neurogenic inflammation, endothelial function, and calcium homeostasis
		ADRA2B	
		ANKDD1B	
		KIAA0040	
Hautakangas et al., 2021 [112]	MA	HMOX2	Inflammation (vascular)
		CACNA1A	Voltage-dependent calcium channel (neurogenic)
		MPPED2	Metalloproteinase
	MO	SPINK2	Protease inhibitor
		FECH	Ferrochelatase

Finally, the largest and most recent meta-analysis on migraine was conducted by Hautakangas et al. [112] in 2022, which included 102,084 migraine cases and 771,257 controls. The team identified three variants associated with MA as follows: (1) rs12598836 in HMOX2, (2) rs10405121 in CACNA1A, and (3) rs11031122 in MPPED2. HMOX2 is a constitutive gene that plays a role in heme catabolism, leading to antioxidant and anti-inflammatory effects [117]. CACNA1A encodes the alpha-1a subunit of the voltage-dependent P/Q calcium channel, and has been linked repeatedly to familial hemiplegic migraine (FHM), a subtype of MA [118]. Finally, MPPED2 is a metallophosphoesterase domain-containing protein which has been linked to various functions, including tumor suppression [119]. On the other hand, the meta-analysis suggested two variants associated with MO as follows: (1) rs7684253 in the locus near SPINK2, a serine peptidase inhibitor, and (2) rs8087942 in the locus near FECH, responsible for the synthesis of ferrochelatase.

At first, GWAS results seemed paradoxical, mainly because the results of these studies showed a more robust genetic association in MO [107], which is contradictory to the results from twin studies and population studies (showing that migraine with aura is more genetic). One possible explanation is that GWAS detects mainly variants with moderate or high allele frequencies (≥ 0.05); thus, relatively rarer alleles cannot be detected. Consequently, experts hypothesize that these rare alleles could be responsible for the genetic susceptibility of MA. As a result, researchers adopted RNA and exome/genome sequencing approaches to assess the contribution of such variants [3].

3.4. Fine Mapping of Potential Migraine Susceptible SNPs

Research was not limited to identifying possible SNPs using GWAS or other techniques. Instead, these potential loci were studied further using various methods. It is important to know that many of the SNPs correlated to migraine have unclear mechanisms of action. Thus, the fine mapping of these potential loci is of great value for understanding the genetics and pathophysiology of migraine. This approach occurs as follows: (1) association-test statistics are used to prioritize a set of SNPs that would likely contain disease-causing SNPs, (2) connecting these variants with genes using resources such as the Encyclopedia of DNA Elements (ENCODE), NIH Roadmap Epigenomics, and FANTOM5, and (3) conducting functional experiments to discern the exact pathophysiological mechanism of this variant/allele [6]. For example, the relationship of PHACTR1 to migraine has been investigated, and the pathophysiological mechanism has been suggested. After rs9349379 has been correlated to migraine (step 1), it was found to be on intron 3 of the PHACTR1 gene (step 2) [109]. Using the CRISPR-edited stem cell-derived endothelial cells, they demonstrated that this SNP regulates the endothelin 1 gene (EDN1), which is located 600 kb upstream of PHACTR1 and encodes a protein that promotes vasoconstriction, extracellular matrix production, fibrosis, and vascular smooth muscle cell proliferation (step 3) [120].

3.5. RNA Sequencing and Transcriptomic Studies

As discussed, GWAS detects high-frequency alleles exclusively, thus, rare variations that give insight into the genetics of migraine are not pinned by these studies. This problem was solved by using more specific techniques such as RNA sequencing and transcriptomic studies. To prevent the capturing bias, researchers have adopted RNA sequencing as a method to investigate migraine genetics. This technique allows investigators to identify novel transcripts, research the role of alternative splicing and gene fusion, and quantify the gene expression level related to migraine [121]. The final goal was also met using transcriptomic methods [41]. Table 6 summarizes studies in which RNA sequencing or transcriptomic studies were adapted.

Table 6. Summary of studies using RNA sequencing and transcriptomic studies.

Articles	Phenotype	Genes	Pathways
Perry et al., 2016 [41] (Transcriptomic study)	Migraine	IL6	
		SOCS3 IFNB CXCR4 CCL2 NFKBIA	Inflammatory pathway
Renthal et al., 2018 [122]	Migraine	CACNA1A SCN1A NOTCH3	Ion channels
Starobova et al., 2018 [123]	Pain	Neuropeptide Y SCN9A SNC10A SCN11A	Ion channels

Table 6. Cont.

Articles	Phenotype	Genes	Pathways
Perry et al., 2016 [41] (Transcriptomic study)	Migraine	IL6 SOCS3 IFNB CXCR4 CCL2 NFKBIA	Inflammatory pathway
Renthal et al., 2018 [122]	Migraine	CACNA1A SCN1A NOTCH3	Ion channels
Starobova et al., 2018 [123]	Pain	Neuropeptide Y SCN9A SNC10A SCN11A	Ion channels
Jeong et al., 2018 [124]	Migraine	LRRC8 WSCD1	Immune response, glutamate signaling pathway, and reactive oxygen species regulation
Kogelman et al., 2019 [125]	MA	NMNAT2 RETN	Unknown
Vgontzas et al., 2020 [126]	MA, MO	HCK ARHGEF26 WSCD1 TSPAN2 NEGR1 SLC24A3 GPR182 NOTCH4 MYO1A HELLS	Central Nervous System Neurovascular cells Peripheral Nervous System
Kogelman et al., 2021 [127]	MA, MO	CPT1A SLC25A20 ETFDH MAML2 ADAM15 ADAM17 CARD9 SH2D2A CD300C	Fatty acid oxidation Notch signaling pathways Immune-related pathways

Renthal et al. (2018) [122] studied single-brain cell RNA sequencing data from cortical cells (neurons, oligodendrocytes, astrocytes, microglia, and endothelial cells). The analysis indicated that 70% and 30% of neuronal migraine-associated genes are significantly enriched in inhibitory and excitatory neurons, respectively, considering that many genes (such as SCN1A and CACNA1A) are found in both neuron types. Additionally, the study showed that 40% of known migraine-associated genes are enriched in a specific brain cell type. Vgontzas et al. (2020) [126] studied single-cell RNA sequencing data from the central and peripheral nervous system (neurons, glial cells, neurovascular cells). They showed that 11.1% of migraine-associated genes were selectively enriched in the central nervous system (HCK, ARHGEF26, WSCD1, TSPAN2, NEGR1, SLC24A3), 5.5% in neurovascular cells (i.e., GPR182, NOTCH4), and 3.7% in the peripheral nervous system (MYO1A, HELLS). Kogelman et al. performed RNA sequencing from the venous blood of MO and MA patients [125]. In 2019, the group compared 17 MO and 9 MA female patients to 20 female controls, and they showed that the genes NMNAT2 and RETN are differentially expressed in MA patients when compared to the controls; however, these results were not replicated in an independent cohort. In 2021 [127], the group compared the gene expression in MA and MO patients during the attack and after treatment. Results showed that 33 genes are differentially expressed between the two phases of migraine; most of these genes play a role in fatty acid oxidation (CPT1A, SLC25A20, and ETFDH), immune-related pathways (CARD9, SH2D2A, CD300C), and notch signaling pathways (MAML2, ADAM15, and ADAM17). Perry et al. [41] conducted a transcriptomic study of the expression of inflammation and immune response genes in chronic migraine patients' calvarial periosteum. They found that 26 genes were upregulated and 11 genes were downregulated. The upregulated genes were associated with the activation of leukocytes, the production of cytokines, and the inhibition of NF-kB, while the downregulated genes were associated with the prevention of macrophage activation and cell lysis. The genes correlated to the pathophysiology of the periosteum are IL6, SOCS3, IFNB, CXCR4, CCL2, and NFKBIA.

3.6. Whole Exome or Whole Genome Sequencing (WES or WGS)

WES reveals nucleotide sequences in the coding region of the DNA, or the exon. WGS is more inclusive as it detects nucleotide sequences in both the coding and non-coding regions of the DNA (exons and introns). Applying the latter technique is important to identify the polymorphisms in the introns that might be responsible for migraine manifestation.

Ibrahim et al. completed whole exome sequencing on 16 individuals with no mutations in the FHM gene [128]. They associated ATP10A (p.Ala881Val) and ATP7B (p. Leu795Phe) variants with migraine. ATP10A encodes an ATPase with flippase activity on plasma membrane lipids, and ATP7B encodes transmembrane copper transporters. Interestingly, the ATP10A is found on locus 15q11-q13, which was pinned in 2005 by Russo et al. [95] using linkage studies (described previously). Additionally, the team suggested the possibility of CACNA1C (p.Ile662Leu) and CACNA1I (p.Arg111Gly) influence [128]. These genes encode voltage-gated calcium channels, similar to CACN1A1, which was pinned in FHM and MA (using GWAS). Another project detected the genes ATXN1 (contributes to glutamate signaling), FAM153B, and CACNA1B (voltage-gated calcium channels) in a population of 620 migraineurs [129,130]. This study was also replicated in 1930 migraine patients, and the same genes were detected. This work represents a combination of GWAS and RNA sequencing. However, it is important to mention that WES or WGS are expensive techniques that come with the burden of increased cost. They also impose some storage burden, which might affect the data quality [74]. In addition, these techniques might result in a capturing bias. For instance, WES is ineffective in capturing all mutations, particularly structural variants such as repetitive regions [131]. Also, migraine susceptibility loci are not limited to coding regions; many loci are in non-coding genomic regions that regulate splicing patterns or downstream genes [132]. Table 7 shows the genes hypothesized to be associated with migraine using WES/WGS.

Table 7. Summary of whole exome and whole genome sequencing studies (WES and WGS).

Article	Phenotype	Genes	Pathway
Williams et al., 2019 [42] (WES and WGS)	Migraine	ALPK1	Centrosome cilia functions Immune response and inflammation
Rasmussen et al., 2020 [129,130] (WGS and RNA seq)	MA/MO	ATXN1	Glutamate signaling
		FAM153B CACNA1B	Voltage-gated calcium channel
Ibrahim et al., 2020 [128] (WES)	Migraine	ATP10A ATP7B	ATPase
		CACNA1C CACNA1I	Voltage-gated calcium channel

3.7. Other Techniques

RT-PCR has been used on animal and cell models by Royal et al. [133] to study migraine genetics. The team studied two variants of the TRESK protein, a K+ channel encoded by the KCNK18 gene. These two variants are TRESK-MT and TRESK-C110R, which are non-functional variants of the potassium channel. Both were associated with migraine; however, only the TRESK-MT variant was shown to correlate with the MA phenotype, leading to the hyperexcitability of trigeminal neurons. The reason for this association is that TRESK-MT produces another variant, the TRESK-MT2, which co-assembles with TREK1 and TREK2, two other K+ channels, and inhibits them. Additionally, miRNA has been demonstrated to play a role in migraine pathophysiology [134,135]. miR-34a-5p and miR-382-5p have been shown to upregulate acutely during migraine attacks (both MO and MA); these markers were found in the blood and in cerebrospinal fluid (CSF), respectively [134]. Similarly, Tafuri et al. [135] showed that miRNA-27b was upregulated and miRNA-181a, miRNA-let-7b, and miRNA-22 were downregulated in MO patients when compared to healthy controls.

4. Monogenic Syndromes

The largest effect of migraine genetics was implied from rare monogenic syndromes with migraine symptoms. Such syndromes present as a set of symptoms, including migraine. As such, researchers correlated the genes mutated in those monogenic syndromes to migraine, which helped investigate the pathophysiological mechanism behind different types of migraine. Examples of these monogenic syndromes are included below.

4.1. CADASIL

Cerebral autosomal dominant arteriopathy with subcortical infarcts and leukoencephalopathy (CADASIL) is an inherited disease caused by a mutation in the *NOTCH3* gene found on chromosome 19. This gene encodes for a transmembrane receptor exclusively restricted to human vascular myocytes [136]. Histopathological studies of vascular tissue in CADASIL patients suggest the thickening and alteration of standard physiologic structure throughout the body [137]; however, the cerebral vasculature seems to be responsible for the majority of the disorder's symptoms, usually including migraine, as the first presenting sign of the disease [136]. Interestingly, a study conducted by Tan et al. [138] showed that more than 75% of 300 symptomatic CADASIL patients experienced migraine, which were accompanied by auras approximately 90% of the time. However, other studies indicate different numbers.

Nevertheless, taking all of the results together, migraine prevalence in CADASIL patients would be around 38%, which is still higher than the general population [138]. Several mechanisms have been proposed to explain the increased prevalence of migraine with auras in CADASIL patients as compared to the general population. One such mechanism centers around the idea that episodic ischemia generated by the vascular changes in the disease could be responsible for a more pronounced cerebral hypoperfusion phase, leading to cerebral blood flow changes similar to those observed in CSD [139], and thereby accounting for more severe auras [140]. Other plausible mechanisms include the possibility that the vascular abnormalities in CADASIL patients could decrease the threshold for CSD, as demonstrated in mice with mutated or deleted NOTCH3 genes [141], that the brainstem involvement in the disease process in CADASIL patients increases their susceptibility for migraine with auras, or that the NOTCH3 gene is involved in the pathway of migraine auras, since genetic studies have shown that family members of migraine patients have an increased risk of experiencing migraine themselves [44,142].

4.2. D-CAA

Cerebral amyloid angiopathy (CAA) is a cerebrovascular disease characterized by the accumulation of β-amyloid molecules in the leptomeninges of the central nervous system and the cerebral vessels [143]. This disease can lead to a severe intracerebral hemorrhage (ICH) in elderly patients [144]. However, preceding the ICH symptoms, migraine with aura often manifests as a presenting sign and an early marker of hereditary cases of CAA, especially Dutch-type CAA (D-CAA). This was seen in a study conducted by Koemans et al. [145], which found a 56% prevalence of migraine with aura in 86 recruited D-CAA patients. Interestingly, migraine was the initial symptom in approximately 80% of the cases [145]. As is the case with other cerebrovascular angiopathies, the exact mechanism behind the onset of migraine in this type of disease is not very well understood. However, several similar theories to the ones mentioned previously have also been suggested.

4.3. COL4A1-Related Disorders

COL4A1 is a gene located on chromosome 13 that encodes for the α-1 subunit of type IV collagen. This subunit plays an important role in the basement membrane of several different tissues in the body, especially the vascular tissue surrounding the blood vessels. Mutations of this gene cause a COL4A1-related brain small-vessel disease, which targets fragile vessels; this leads to hereditary infantile hemiparesis, retinal arteriolar tortuosity and leukoencephalopathy, and familial porencephaly [146,147]. Several studies show that migraine with aura may be a symptom of this mutation, as presented in a study of six affected family members, where 50% presented with auras [148]. This is also seen in a systematic review conducted by Lanfranconi et al. [149], in which 10 out of 52 carrier subjects had experienced migraine.

4.4. FASPS

Familial advanced sleep-phase syndrome (FASPS) is an autosomal dominant disorder caused by a missense mutation in the CSNK1D gene, which encodes for the Casein Kinase Iδ (CK1δ) [150], a serine/threonine kinase which phosphorylates several important target proteins in order to regulate the cell cycle, cell differentiation, proliferation, and the circadian clock [151,152]. Patients usually experience an earlier sleep onset and morning awakening, often described as "morning larks" [153]. Interestingly, in two different mutations (T44A and H46R) of the CSNK1D gene in transgenic mice, a co-segregation was also found with MA [150,154,155]. In essence, sensitization to pain resulting from nitroglycerin-triggered migraine reduced the threshold for CSD, and increased calcium signaling were detected in the T44A transgenic mice [150,155], thus explaining the co-presence of MA with the disease. Involved in migraine pathogenesis, the CSNK1D gene provides evidence for the involvement of the hypothalamus in the development of and susceptibility to migraine.

4.5. KCNK18

The TWIK-related spinal cord potassium channel (TRESK) is a member of the two-pore domain potassium (K2P) channel family—an important modulator of the resting membrane potential—encoded by the KCNK18 gene [156]. A frameshift mutation in this gene produces a truncated and non-functional channel, which can also suppress the levels of the wild-type channel and increase the susceptibility to migraine with aura [157]. This mutation was first discovered in a patient suffering from MA, and was later also confirmed in seven of the patient's relatives who also suffered from the same disease [156].

4.6. ROSAH Syndrome

Heterozygous missense variants of the α-kinase gene ALPK1 are responsible for the pathogenesis of ROSAH syndrome, named after its five main symptoms: retinal dystrophy, optic nerve edema, splenomegaly, anhidrosis, and migraine headache [42]. This gene has been detected at high levels in the retina, in the retinal pigment epithelium, and in the optic nerve. It is important to note that migraine is also a frequent feature of the disease.

4.7. HERNS

Hereditary endotheliopathy with retinopathy, nephropathy, and stroke (HERNS) is an autosomal dominant systemic multi-infarct disorder that was first described by

Jen et al. [158] in 1997 in a Chinese American family. As its name implies, this disease first manifests as visual impairment due to macular edema and as renal dysfunction with albuminuria [158]. The neurologic symptoms usually appear in the second decade of life, most commonly emerging as migraine headaches, in addition to psychiatric manifestations, hemiparesis, dysarthria, and others [158,159]. The mechanism behind the disease is generalized vascular damage in different capillaries and arterioles of the body, including retinal, cerebral, and renal areas [158,160].

4.8. MELAS

Mitochondrial encephalopathy, lactic acidosis, and stroke-like episodes (MELAS) syndromes are most commonly caused by an A to g transition mutation at position 3243 of the mitochondrial genome [161,162]. It is characterized by recurrent attacks of migraine-like headaches with vomiting, epilepsy, and stroke-like episodes, accompanied with blindness, deafness, cognitive impairment, and cardiac conduction defects, among others [163–166]. Even though the transition cited previously is the primary mutation seen in MELAS, it is, however, a polygenic disease caused by several mutations that involve mitochondrial tRNA and protein-coding genes, some of which are also involved in other mitochondrial diseases, such as LHON, Leigh Disease, and MERRF [167]. However, surprisingly, studies performed by Buzzi and colleagues [168] and Cevoli et al. [169] on maternal lineages with MELAS showed that most subjects were monosymptomatic, with the disease manifesting only as migraine. In addition, all of the migraine-only subjects did not carry the 3243 A > G tRNA Leu (MELAS) mutation, suggesting that this mutation does not contribute to the maternal multigenerational migraine with or without aura [168].

4.9. RVCL-S

Retinal vasculopathy with cerebral leukoencephalopathy and systemic manifestations (RVCL-S) is a rare systemic small-vessel disease caused by an autosomal dominant mutation in the three-prime repair exonuclease 1 (TREX1), mainly affecting the white matter of the CNS [170,171]. The amyloid-negative angiopathy involves mostly small vessels such as arterioles and capillaries in several locations of the body, including the retina and the brain [172]. This disorder is characterized by retinopathy, neurological deficits, and other systemic symptoms, including anemia, liver disease, kidney injury, and Raynaud's phenomenon [170]. Migraine with and without aura are sometimes also reported by affected patients, as reported by 42% of patients in cross-sectional studies [172–175]. These kinds of migraine tend to occur in adult RVCL-S patients, compared to the earlier onset (childhood or adolescence) in the general population, which could suggest that vasculopathy is responsible for the onset of the migraine in these patients [175].

4.10. CCM

Familial cerebral cavernous malformations (CCM) is a heritable autosomal dominant disease characterized by at least three mutations in three different loci as follows: CCM1 on chromosome 7q, CCM2 on chromosome 7p, and CCM3 on chromosome 3p, characterized by vascular abnormalities in the central nervous system (CNS), leading to epileptic seizures and hemorrhagic strokes [176–179]. Several studies have also found migraine to be a symptom of this disorder [179].

5. Familial Hemiplegic Migraine (FHM)

As discussed, familial hemiplegic migraine (FHM) represents a rare autosomal dominant subtype of MA with an obligatory presence of a motor aura, represented by reversible motor weakness—hence the "hemiplegic" part of the disease—that is most often, but not always, unilateral [180,181]. Additionally, the diagnostic guidelines of the third edition of the International Classification of Headache Disorders, provided by the Headache Classification Committee of the International Headache Society, require the presence of at least one first- or second-degree relative having a migraine with motor auras (Table 8) [11]. The age interval of clinical appearances is flexible, stretching from 5 to 30 years old in most cases, with migraine tending to appear more in younger people [182]. Aside from the essential motor aura symptoms, a population-based study by Thomsen et al. showed that the other most common aura types were sensory, visual, and aphasia [183]. Even though motor, sensory, and visual auras were essentially similar to those seen in MA, their duration was significantly longer in FHM than in MA [180]. Many trigger factors have been implicated in the appearance of FHM, including acute stress, emotional fluctuation, excess or lack of sleep, minor head trauma, and menstruation in women [184–186]. In addition, more than two-thirds of FHM patients displayed a co-occurrence of basilar migraine (BM) as well, defined according to the IHS guidelines [183]. An overlap between epilepsy and migraine has also been suggested by the presence of seizures in certain specific pathogenic cases of FHM [187,188]. Being genetically heterogeneous, FHM has been divided into three subtypes, based on the genetic mutation responsible for the disease presentation (Figure 2).

Table 8. ICHD criteria for familial hemiplegic migraine diagnosis [11].

A.	Fulfilling hemiplegic migraine criteria	1. Attacks fulfilling the criteria for migraine with aura (Table 1).
		 2. Aura consisting of <u>both</u> of the following:
		    2.1. fully reversible motor weakness,
		    2.2. fully reversible visual, sensory, and/or speech/language symptoms.

B.	At least one first- or second-degree relative who experienced attacks fulfilling criteria in "A".	

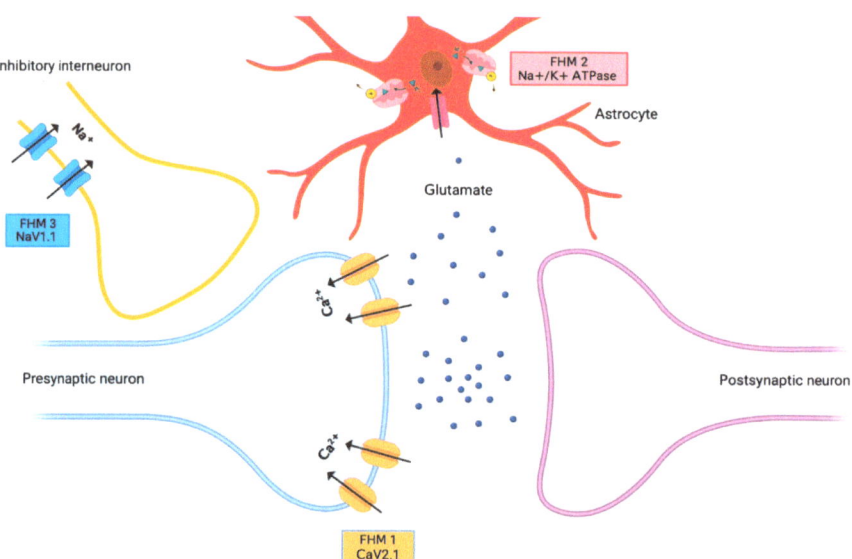

Figure 2. Figure representing the channels inhibited by each type of familial hemiplegic migraine.

5.1. FHM1

Familial hemiplegic migraine type 1 (FHM1) was first identified to be related to a specific genetic mutation in 1996, when Ophoff et al. demonstrated the presence of a CACNA1A mutation on chromosome 19p13. This gene encodes the pore-forming α1 subunit of the P/Q type calcium channel CaV2.1, which is found on presynaptic and somatodendritic membranes [21,189]. In fact, the study found four missense mutations associated with the presentation of the disease. However, several other mutations have been added to the list [190,191].

5.1.1. Calcium Channels

As indicated by Bolay et al. [8], the most plausible and acceptable mechanism of migraine auras today is an increased cortical spreading depression (CSD) in the brain; genetic mutations in the aforementioned trio of genes are linked with augmented concentrations of neurotransmitters and potassium ions at the synaptic cleft, which may cause the cortical spreading depression commonly seen in migraine aura [192]. Contemporary studies that have physiologically induced visual auras have implicated cortical spreading depression in the onset of a migraine aura, which is accompanied by symptoms such as visual, language, or motor impairments [193]. Although the etiology of a migraine aura remained highly debated, understanding the involvement of specific channels may provide valuable insights. In recent studies involving mice, those with R192Q or S218L missense mutants in the α1 subunit of the Cav2.1 Ca2+ channels exhibited spontaneous cortical spreading depression events (CSD); mutant mice had a reduced threshold and a greater propagation speed for these events, which align with FHM1 clinical phenotypes [194]. The role of CaV2.1 channel activity in CSD has been thoroughly investigated by Ayata et al. [195] using in vivo cortical microdialysis on leaner and tottering mice, with tg^{la} and tg mutations in the α1A subunit of CaV2.1, respectively. These mutations have been shown to decrease the density of Ca2+ currents significantly and increase the activation threshold of CaV2.1 channels, thereby reducing the probability of their activation when compared to wild-type mice [196]. In essence, the previously mentioned in vivo studies showed a two-fold reduction in glutamate release in the mutant mice as compared to the wild type and a 10-fold increase in the resistance to CSD following KCl-induction and electrical stimulation [195]. As such, these findings support the assumption that a decreased Ca2+ influx through the CaV2.1 channels increases the resistance to CSD, hence decreasing the plausibility of an aura. Therefore, it would be logical to assume that the mutations seen in FHM1 should have an opposite gain-of-function effect to increase the susceptibility of CSD in patients.

5.1.2. Specific Mutations

A study conducted by van den Maagdenberg et al. [197] on knockin transgenic mice models with the R192Q human mutation responsible for FHM1 found that CaV2.1 channels in the mutant mice open more rapidly and have a lower activation threshold, thereby opening at lower potentials when compared to wild-type channels. In addition, the current density through the mutant CaV2.1 channels was higher than that in wild-type channels, and neurotransmission at the synapses was also increased through an elevated neuromuscular junction concentration of glutamate with approximately constant concentrations of GABA, an inhibitory neurotransmitter [197]. Other studies also showed that the increased contribution of these P/Q calcium channels causes an increase in the release of glutamate by cortical neurons at physiologic microtubule Ca2+ levels [198]. These findings support the previously stated hypothesis that FHM1 results from gain-of-function mutations of the CaV2.1 channels, leading to a reduced threshold for the CSD. This was further supported by Eikermann-Haerter and colleagues [199], who showed that mutant mice with the same R192Q mutation had an elevated frequency of CSD and an increased speed of propagation following KCl induction stimulation studies. Even though R192Q mutant mice expressed pure FHM1 symptoms with hemiplegia only, S218L, another studied mutation in the same knockin mice, showed a more severe phenotype, characterized by seizures, cerebellar symptoms, coma, and possibly fatal cerebral edema occurring after minor head trauma due to more severe calcium channel dysfunction [197,199]. In addition, further studies showed that the underlying mechanism for the phenotypic differences between these two mutations is the level of the subcortical spread of the depression, in such a way that the spread is limited to the striatum only in the R192Q mutations, but more diffused to involve the hippocampus and the thalamus in the S218L mutation [200]. Thus, being highly susceptible to CSD, FHM1 patients develop more severe and prolonged hemiplegic auras. Motor deficits were significantly more prolonged (around 20 more minutes) in these FHM1 mutant mice when compared to the wild type [199].

5.2. FHM2

The gene responsible for the familial hemiplegic migraine type 2 (FHM2) was first identified in 2003 when the gene encoding the α2 subunit, the Na+/K+ ATPase, in neurons and astrocytes—ATP1A2 gene of chromosome 1q23—was discovered in two Italian families [201]. In essence, four α subunits have been identified for the Na+/K+ ATPase [202,203], with the testis-specific α4 subunit and the ubiquitous α1 subunit expressing no pathological mutations. However, the neuron-specific α3 subunit and the astrocyte-specific α2 subunit demonstrate mutations that cause neurological manifestations, essentially rapid-onset dystonia Parkinsonism and FHM2, respectively [204,205]. A more recent case study featuring a male adolescent who was diagnosed with familial hemiplegic migraine (FHM2) revealed a heterozygous genetic mutation within the ATP1A2 gene (c.1133C > T); this missense mutation may inhibit the function of the α2 subunit of the Na+/K+ ATPase [206].

5.2.1. Na+/K+ ATPase

Na+/K+ ATPase pumps are essential for maintaining the resting membrane potential in neurons [207] and generating an ion gradient that is needed for neurotransmitter and nutrient uptake by the cells. As for the glial- and neuron-specific Na+/K+ ATPase pumps, they play an important role in clearing K+ ions from the synaptic cleft after neuronal transmission, a clearance that follows an initial fast phase and a late slow phase by driving K+ ions into the cells, while extruding Na+ ions to the outside [208,209]. This process is essential for the reuptake of glutamate from the synaptic cleft, which is mostly performed via the Na+-dependent glutamate uptake transporters primarily expressed in astrocytes [210,211]. Also, an actual physical association has been suggested linking this Na+/K+ ATPase subunit to glutamate transporters [212], and this was further asserted by an approximately identical localization of the α2 subunit of this Na+/K+ ATPase and glutamate transporters GLAST and GLUT1 in the somatosensory cortex of rats [213]. Hence, it would be logical to assume that the FHM2 mutations should be loss-of-function mutations, keeping high glutamate and/or K+ levels in the synaptic cleft, which can increase the susceptibility to CSD. The involvement of both α2 and α3 subunits of the Na+/K+ ATPase pumps in CSD has been shown in hippocampal slices, where the administration of ouabain, an inhibitor of the Na+/K+ ATPase, at concentrations that have minimal effects on the α1 subunit, significantly reduced the induction threshold for CSD via y increasing the extracellular levels of K+ [214].

5.2.2. Specific Mutations

Several different mutations have been implicated in the pathogenesis of the disease, most of them being missense mutations [215–218]. Two specific mutations, W887R and L764P, have been shown to cause a loss of function in the Na+/K+ ATPase pumps, demonstrated by the inhibition of their currents while maintaining their plasma membrane expressions, suggesting the inactivation of these channels [219]. Other mutations, such as T345A, R689Q, and M731T, have normal function but altered kinetics, demonstrated by a decreased catalytic turnover and an increased affinity for extracellular K+ [220,221]. A study conducted by Leo et al. [222] generated knockin mice with the human W887R mutation responsible for FHM2. As expected, homozygous mutations were lethal. This was attributed to selective apoptosis in the amygdala and piriform cortex in response to the neuronal hyperactivity and to a depression of the brainstem reticular formation activity, demonstrated by an abolished respiration [223,224].

On the other hand, heterozygous mutations allowed for viable mice with a hypercontractile heart [225]. In essence, the study showed that, even though the mutant R887 allele is correctly transcribed and translated, it is sequestered by the endoplasmic reticulum and proteasome system, inhibiting its expression on the cell surface, in contrast to previous findings [222]. In vivo electrical cortical stimulation showed an increased susceptibility of the mutant mice to CSD when compared to the wild type, demonstrated through a decreased induction threshold and a higher propagation velocity [222]. This is most probably due to an accumulation of K+ in the synaptic cleft above physiological ranges, due to a decrease in the number and/or the activity of the α2 subunit of Na+/K+ ATPases in astrocytes, leading to a constant stimulation of the nervous system, eventually advancing to a CSD [181]. Other mutations were also noted in a large clinical investigation, comprising FHM2 patients alongside their clinical manifestations. Those with pure FHM had R65W, R202Q, R593W, and T762S variants in the ATP1A2 gene. Conversely, those with FHM and epilepsy displayed mutations such as R548C, E825K, and R928P in this gene. Individuals with FHM accompanied by epilepsy and intellectual disabilities harbored the T378N, G615R, and D718N mutants [226].

5.3. FHM3

Familial hemiplegic migraine type 3 (FHM3) was linked to a specific gene in 2005 after discovering a mutation in the SCN1A gene on chromosome 2q24 in three German families [227]. This gene encodes the α1 pore-forming subunit of the voltage-gated Na+ channel NaV1.1.

5.3.1. Voltage-Gated Sodium Channels NaV1.1

The expression of NaV1.1 channels peaks during the third postnatal week, and then decreases dramatically to approximately half its peak expression in adult life. It is most likely localized to the brainstem, cortex, substantia nigra, and the caudate nucleus, as indicated by studies on adult rat brains [228]. These channels are mostly concentrated in the somatodendritic area, especially in hippocampal, pyramidal, and inhibitory neurons [229]. A study conducted by Yu et al. [230] showed that heterozygous and homozygous loss-of-function mutations of the SCN1A gene in Scn1a$^{+/-}$ and Scn1a$^{-/-}$ mice, respectively, experienced a decreased sodium current intensity in inhibitory GABAergic neurons, without any significant effect on excitatory neurons in the brain. Even though homozygous mice experienced ataxia and died on the 15th postnatal day, heterozygous mice suffered from seizures that led to severe myoclonic epilepsy in infancy (SMEI), and most were killed by the 21st postnatal day [230]. In essence, these findings suggest that the decreased sodium currents through mutant NaV1.1 channels in GABAergic neurons led to a decrease in GABA release throughout the nervous system. This phenomenon resulted in hyperexcitability responsible for the generation of seizures and epilepsies in affected mice. A study conducted by Gargus et al. [231] confirmed that the SCN1A gene known to be responsible for SMEI is, in fact, the exact gene responsible for the onset of FHM3. Thus, one would assume that a similar mechanism could also be found in FHM3 mutant NaV1.1 channels, where hyperexcitability could potentiate the appearance of CSD.

5.3.2. Specific Mutations

Even though a loss-of-function mutation was expected to be responsible for the pathogenesis of the migraine, as previously observed in the appearance of SMEI [230], FHM3 proved to result from gain-of-function mutations [232–234]. Jansen and colleagues [235] generated the first transgenic mouse model for FHM3 expressing the L263V mutation. The excessive firing of inhibitory GABAergic neurons could increase CSD susceptibility via increasing extracellular K+ concentrations [236]. In addition, Wiwanitkit [237] found that the FHM3 protein is more resistant than both FHM1 and FHM2.3.1.

5.4. FHM4

Even though the involvement of three genes has been established in the onset of FHM, new research suggests the involvement of a fourth gene, PRRT2, in the rise of familial hemiplegic migraine. A novel case study featured a Portuguese patient with a heterozygous missense mutation (c.938C > T;p.Ala313Val), which inhibits the protein's stability and subcellular localization [238]. In another study, a 13-year-old FHM patient who harbored a microdeletion in the chromosome 16p11.2 loci displayed a haploinsufficiency for the PRRT2 gene, which encodes a proline-rich transmembrane protein [239]. Further research studies are necessary to further elucidate the involvement of this gene in FHM; however, these physiological consequences indicate that the PRRT2 gene may be the fourth gene involved in the pathogenesis of FHM.

5.4.1. PRRT2 Protein

The PRRT2 protein is vital in proper neuronal development, healthy synaptic formation, and the release of neurotransmitters into the synaptic cleft. A variety of mutations in this gene, such as missense or deletions, has resulted in haploinsufficiency, which can be associated with various diseases, such as FHM or benign familial infantile epilepsy (BFIE) [240]. This protein is localized within the cortical layers of several neurological structures, such as the cerebral cortex, and may play a role in negatively modulating the Nav1.2 and Nav1.6 Na+ channels; mutations in this gene have led to hyperexcitability and an increased Na+ current in mutated neurons [241]. Thus, this protein is vital in maintaining neuronal network stability. A loss of function in this gene may be associated with synaptic deregulation or a decrease in the number of synapses, neuronal hyperexcitability, and the inhibition of the synchronous release of neurotransmitters by affected neurons [242].

5.4.2. Specific Mutations

A genetic variant in the PRRT2 gene (NM_145239.3:c.938C > T; p.Ala313Val) was discovered via a WES family analysis in a 40-year-old male patient suffering from migraine with aura [243]. A physiological consequence of this missense mutation is disrupted protein stability; alterations in amino acid polarity impact the chemical dynamic between neighboring residues, which alters the three-dimensional folding of the protein. In another clinical study, twenty-two FHM patients from four families exhibited mutations in the PRRT2 gene as follows: c.649_650insC, c.649dupC, c.843C > G, and c.649dupC. Though limited, these studies indicate that mutations in the PRRT2 gene may be a genetic mechanism for hemiplegic migraine; however, further studies are needed to thoroughly examine the role of this gene [243].

6. Conclusions

It is crucial to study the history of migraine genetics and refer back to previously adapted techniques in its study. MA/MO genetics was studied initially using population and twin studies to learn about their heritability; then, many genetic techniques were used, including CGAS, GWAS, linkage studies, exome/genome sequencing, and RNA sequencing. Different loci were correlated to migraine using these techniques, with some of them pinned using more than one technique. Additionally, monogenic syndromes played a major role in identifying the genes responsible for migraine genetics. This review summarizes the major findings of the techniques used to study MO/MA genetics since its dawn. Additionally, great work has been completed to discern the genes responsible for FHM and SHM; we discussed the identified genes and their pathophysiological mechanisms which could be referred to for further reference. The study of migraine genetics has its limitations, including the diversity of techniques and results. Further studies are needed to advance this field further and decrease the ambiguities.

Author Contributions: Conceptualization, M.A. and K.T.; methodology, M.A., K.T., N.G.Z., E.S., J.M.K. and E.G.; writing—original draft preparation, M.A., K.T., N.G.Z., E.S., J.M.K. and E.G.; writing—review and editing, M.A., K.T., N.G.Z., E.S., J.M.K. and E.G.; supervision, M.A. and K.T. All authors have read and agreed to the published version of the manuscript.

Funding: This research received no external funding.

Data Availability Statement: No new data were gathered or analyzed. Data sharing is not applicable to this paper.

Conflicts of Interest: The authors declare no conflicts of interest.

Abbreviations

MA	Migraine with aura
MO	Migraine without aura
FHM	Familial hemiplegic migraine
CSD	Cortical spreading depression
ICHD-3	International Classification of Headache Disorders-3
CGAS	Candidate-gene association studies
LCA	Latent class analysis
TCA	Trait component analysis
GWAS	Genome-wide association study
MTHFR	Methylenetetrahydrofolate reductase

References

1. Headache Classification Committee of the International Headache Society (IHS). The International Classification of Headache Disorders, 3rd edition. *Cephalalgia* **2018**, *38*, 1–211. [CrossRef]
2. de Boer, I.; Terwindt, G.M.; van den Maagdenberg, A. Genetics of migraine aura: An update. *J. Headache Pain* **2020**, *21*, 64. [CrossRef]
3. de Boer, I.; van den Maagdenberg, A.; Terwindt, G.M. Advance in genetics of migraine. *Curr. Opin. Neurol.* **2019**, *32*, 413–421. [CrossRef]
4. Aguilar-Shea, A.L.; Membrilla Md, J.A.; Diaz-de-Teran, J. Migraine review for general practice. *Aten. Primaria* **2022**, *54*, 102208. [CrossRef]
5. Steiner, T.J.; Stovner, L.J.; Jensen, R.; Uluduz, D.; Katsarava, Z. Migraine remains second among the world's causes of disability, and first among young women: Findings from GBD2019. *J. Headache Pain* **2020**, *21*, 137. [CrossRef]
6. Sutherland, H.G.; Albury, C.L.; Griffiths, L.R. Advances in genetics of migraine. *J. Headache Pain* **2019**, *20*, 72. [CrossRef] [PubMed]
7. Hadjikhani, N.; Sanchez Del Rio, M.; Wu, O.; Schwartz, D.; Bakker, D.; Fischl, B.; Kwong, K.K.; Cutrer, F.M.; Rosen, B.R.; Tootell, R.B.H.; et al. Mechanisms of migraine aura revealed by functional MRI in human visual cortex. *Proc. Natl. Acad. Sci. USA* **2001**, *98*, 4687–4692. [CrossRef] [PubMed]
8. Bolay, H.; Reuter, U.; Dunn, A.K.; Huang, Z.; Boas, D.A.; Moskowitz, M.A. Intrinsic brain activity triggers trigeminal meningeal afferents in a migraine model. *Nat. Med.* **2002**, *8*, 136–142. [CrossRef] [PubMed]
9. Zhang, X.; Levy, D.; Noseda, R.; Kainz, V.; Jakubowski, M.; Burstein, R. Activation of meningeal nociceptors by cortical spreading depression: Implications for migraine with aura. *J. Neurosci.* **2010**, *30*, 8807–8814. [CrossRef]
10. Le, H.; Tfelt-Hansen, P.; Skytthe, A.; Kyvik, K.O.; Olesen, J. Increase in self-reported migraine prevalence in the Danish adult population: A prospective longitudinal population-based study. *BMJ Open* **2012**, *2*, e000962. [CrossRef]
11. Headache Classification Committee of the International Headache Society (IHS). The international classification of headache disorders, (beta version). *Cephalalgia* **2013**, *33*, 629–808. [CrossRef] [PubMed]
12. Schwedt, T.J.; Zhou, J.; Dodick, D.W. Sporadic hemiplegic migraine with permanent neurological deficits. *Headache J. Head. Face Pain* **2014**, *54*, 163–166. [CrossRef] [PubMed]
13. Riant, F.; Ducros, A.; Ploton, C.; Barbance, C.; Depienne, C.; Tournier-Lasserve, E. De novo mutations in ATP1A2 and CACNA1A are frequent in early-onset sporadic hemiplegic migraine. *Neurology* **2010**, *75*, 967–972. [CrossRef] [PubMed]
14. Black, D.F. Sporadic hemiplegic migraine. *Curr. Pain Headache Rep.* **2004**, *8*, 223–228. [CrossRef] [PubMed]
15. Martínez, E.; Moreno, R.; López-Mesonero, L.; Vidriales, I.; Ruiz, M.; Guerrero, A.; Tellería, J.J. Familial hemiplegic migraine with severe attacks: A new report with ATP1A2 mutation. *Case Rep. Neurol. Med.* **2016**, *2016*, 3464285. [PubMed]
16. Carreño, O.; Corominas, R.; Serra, S.A.; Sintas, C.; Fernández-Castillo, N.; Vila-Pueyo, M.; Toma, C.; Gené, G.G.; Pons, R.; Llaneza, M.; et al. Screening of *CACNA1A* and *ATP1A2* genes in hemiplegic migraine: Clinical, genetic, and functional studies. *Mol. Genet. Genom. Med.* **2013**, *1*, 206–222. [CrossRef] [PubMed]
17. Di Cristofori, A.; Fusi, L.; Gomitoni, A.; Grampa, G.; Bersano, A. R583Q CACNA1A variant in SHM1 and ataxia: Case report and literature update. *J. Headache Pain* **2012**, *13*, 419–423. [CrossRef] [PubMed]
18. De Vries, B.; Freilinger, T.; Vanmolkot, K.R.J.; Koenderink, J.B.; Stam, A.H.; Terwindt, G.M.; Babini, E.; Van Den Boogerd, E.H.; Van Den Heuvel, J.J.M.W.; Frants, R.R.; et al. Systematic analysis of three FHM genes in 39 sporadic patients with hemiplegic migraine. *Neurology* **2007**, *69*, 2170–2176. [CrossRef] [PubMed]
19. Zangaladze, A.; Asadi-Pooya, A.A.; Ashkenazi, A.; Sperling, M.R. Sporadic hemiplegic migraine and epilepsy associated with CACNA1A gene mutation. *Epilepsy Behav.* **2010**, *17*, 293–295. [CrossRef]
20. Jokubaitis, M.; Lengvenis, G.; Burnytė, B.; Audronytė, E.; Ryliškienė, K. Case report: Late onset type 3 hemiplegic migraine with permanent neurologic sequelae after attacks. *Front. Neurol.* **2024**, *15*, 1359994. [CrossRef]

21. Ophoff, R.A.; Terwindt, G.M.; Vergouwe, M.N.; Van Eijk, R.; Oefner, P.J.; Hoffman, S.M.; Lamerdin, J.E.; Mohrenweiser, H.W.; Bulman, D.E.; Ferrari, M. Familial hemiplegic migraine and episodic ataxia type-2 are caused by mutations in the Ca2+ channel gene CACNL1A4. *Cell* 1996, *87*, 543–552. [CrossRef] [PubMed]
22. Russell, M.B.; Ducros, A. Sporadic and familial hemiplegic migraine: Pathophysiological mechanisms, clinical characteristics, diagnosis, and management. *Lancet Neurol.* 2011, *10*, 457–470. [CrossRef] [PubMed]
23. Di Stefano, V.; Rispoli, M.G.; Pellegrino, N.; Graziosi, A.; Rotondo, E.; Napoli, C.; Pietrobon, D.; Brighina, F.; Parisi, P. Diagnostic and therapeutic aspects of hemiplegic migraine. *J. Neurol. Neurosurg. Psychiatry* 2020, *91*, 764–771. [CrossRef] [PubMed]
24. Rasmussen, B.K.; Olesen, J. Migraine with aura and migraine without aura: An epidemiological study. *Cephalalgia* 1992, *12*, 221–228. [CrossRef] [PubMed]
25. Ziegler, D.K.; Hur, Y.-M.; Bouchard, T.J.; Hassanein, R.S.; Barter, R. Migraine in Twins Raised Together and Apart. *Headache J. Head. Face Pain* 1998, *38*, 417–422. [CrossRef] [PubMed]
26. Frosst, P.; Blom, H.J.; Milos, R.; Goyette, P.; Sheppard, C.A.; Matthews, R.G.; Boers, G.J.H.; Den Heijer, M.; Kluijtmans, L.A.J.; Van Den Heuve, L.P.; et al. A candidate genetic risk factor for vascular disease: A common mutation in methylenetetrahydrofolate reductase. *Nat. Genet.* 1995, *10*, 111–113. [CrossRef] [PubMed]
27. Kowa, H.; Yasui, K.; Takeshima, T.; Urakami, K.; Sakai, F.; Nakashima, K. The homozygous C677T mutation in the methylenetetrahydrofolate reductase gene is a genetic risk factor for migraine. *Am. J. Med. Genet.* 2000, *96*, 762–764. [CrossRef] [PubMed]
28. Kara, I.; Sazci, A.; Ergul, E.; Kaya, G.; Kilic, G. Association of the C677T and A1298C polymorphisms in the 5,10 methylenetetrahydrofolate reductase gene in patients with migraine risk. *Brain Res. Mol. Brain Res.* 2003, *111*, 84–90. [CrossRef] [PubMed]
29. Lea, R.A.; Ovcaric, M.; Sundholm, J.; Macmillan, J.; Griffiths, L.R. The methylenetetrahydrofolate reductase gene variant C677T influences susceptibility to migraine with aura. *BMC Med.* 2004, *2*, 3. [CrossRef]
30. Oterino, A.; Valle, N.; Bravo, Y.; Muñoz, P.; Sánchez-Velasco, P.; Ruiz-Alegría, C.; Castillo, J.; Leyva-Cobián, F.; Vadillo, A.; Pascual, J. MTHFR T677 Homozygosis Influences the Presence of Aura in Migraineurs. *Cephalalgia* 2004, *24*, 491–494. [CrossRef]
31. Oterino, A.; Valle, N.; Pascual, J.; Bravo, Y.; Munoz, P.; Castillo, J.; Ruiz-Alegria, C.; Sanchez-Velasco, P.; Leyva-Cobian, F.; Cid, C. Thymidylate synthase promoter tandem repeat and MTHFD1 R653Q polymorphisms modulate the risk for migraine conferred by the MTHFR T677 allele. *Brain Res. Mol. Brain Res.* 2005, *139*, 163–168. [CrossRef] [PubMed]
32. Scher, A.I.; Terwindt, G.M.; Verschuren, W.M.M.; Kruit, M.C.; Blom, H.J.; Kowa, H.; Frants, R.R.; Van Den Maagdenberg, A.M.J.M.; Van Buchem, M.; Ferrari, M.D.; et al. Migraine and MTHFR C677T genotype in a population-based sample. *Ann. Neurol.* 2006, *59*, 372–375. [CrossRef] [PubMed]
33. Rubino, E.; Ferrero, M.; Rainero, I.; Binello, E.; Vaula, G.; Pinessi, L. Association of the C677T polymorphism in the MTHFR gene with migraine: A meta-analysis. *Cephalalgia* 2009, *29*, 818–825. [CrossRef] [PubMed]
34. Liu, R.; Geng, P.; Ma, M.; Yu, S.; Yang, M.; He, M.; Dong, Z.; Zhang, W. MTHFR C677T polymorphism and migraine risk: A meta-analysis. *J. Neurol. Sci.* 2014, *336*, 68–73. [CrossRef] [PubMed]
35. Schürks, M.; Rist, P.M.; Kurth, T. MTHFR677 C>T and ACE D/I Polymorphisms in Migraine: A Systematic Review and Meta-Analysis. *Headache J. Head. Face Pain* 2010, *50*, 588–599. [CrossRef] [PubMed]
36. Samaan, Z.; Gaysina, D.; Cohen-Woods, S.; Craddock, N.; Jones, L.; Korszun, A.; Owen, M.; Mente, A.; McGuffin, P.; Farmer, A. Methylenetetrahydrofolate Reductase Gene Variant (MTHFR C677T) and Migraine: A Case Control Study and Meta-analysis. *BMC Neurol.* 2011, *11*, 66. [CrossRef]
37. Nyholt, D.R.; Curtain, R.P.; Griffiths, L.R. Familial typical migraine: Significant linkage and localization of a gene to Xq24–28. *Hum. Genet.* 2000, *107*, 18–23. [PubMed]
38. Nyholt, D.R.; Morley, K.I.; Ferreira, M.A.R.; Medland, S.E.; Boomsma, D.I.; Heath, A.C.; Merikangas, K.R.; Montgomery, G.W.; Martin, N.G. Genomewide Significant Linkage to Migrainous Headache on Chromosome 5q21. *Am. J. Hum. Genet.* 2005, *77*, 500–512. [CrossRef]
39. Anttila, V.; Kallela, M.; Oswell, G.; Kaunisto, M.A.; Nyholt, D.R.; Hämäläinen, E.; Havanka, H.; Ilmavirta, M.; Terwilliger, J.; Sobel, E.; et al. Trait Components Provide Tools to Dissect the Genetic Susceptibility of Migraine. *Am. J. Hum. Genet.* 2006, *79*, 85–99. [CrossRef] [PubMed]
40. Anttila, V. Genome-wide association study of migraine implicates a common susceptibility variant on 8q22.1. *Nat. Genet.* 2010, *42*, 869–873. [CrossRef]
41. Perry, C.J.; Blake, P.; Buettner, C.; Papavassiliou, E.; Schain, A.J.; Bhasin, M.K.; Burstein, R. Upregulation of inflammatory gene transcripts in periosteum of chronic migraineurs: Implications for extracranial origin of headache. *Ann. Neurol.* 2016, *79*, 1000–1013. [CrossRef] [PubMed]
42. Williams, L.B.; Javed, A.; Sabri, A.; Morgan, D.J.; Huff, C.D.; Grigg, J.R.; Heng, X.T.; Khng, A.J.; Hollink, I.H.; Morrison, M.A. ALPK1 missense pathogenic variant in five families leads to ROSAH syndrome, an ocular multisystem autosomal dominant disorder. *Genet. Med.* 2019, *21*, 2103–2115. [CrossRef] [PubMed]
43. Russell, M.B.; Olesen, J. The genetics of migraine without aura and migraine with aura. *Cephalalgia* 1993, *13*, 245–248. [CrossRef] [PubMed]
44. Russell, M.B.; Olesen, J. Increased familial risk and evidence of genetic factor in migraine. *BMJ* 1995, *311*, 541–544. [CrossRef] [PubMed]
45. Russell, M.; Iselius, L.; Olesen, J. Inheritance of migraine investigated by complex segregation analysis. *Hum. Genet.* 1995, *96*, 726–730. [CrossRef] [PubMed]

46. Stewart, W.F.; Staffa, J.; Lipton, R.B.; Ottman, R. Familial risk of migraine: A population-based study. *Ann. Neurol.* **1997**, *41*, 166–172. [CrossRef] [PubMed]
47. Ulrich, V. The inheritance of migraine with aura estimated by means of structural equation modelling. *J. Med. Genet.* **1999**, *36*, 225–227. [CrossRef] [PubMed]
48. Ulrich, V.; Gervil, M.; Kyvik, K.O.; Olesen, J.; Russell, M.B. Evidence of a genetic factor in migraine with aura: A population-based Danish twin study. *Ann. Neurol.* **1999**, *45*, 242–246. [CrossRef] [PubMed]
49. Waters, W.E.; O'Connor, P.J. Prevalence of migraine. *J. Neurol. Neurosurg. Psychiatry* **1975**, *38*, 613–616. [CrossRef]
50. Gervil, M. Migraine without Aura: A Population-Based Twin Study. *Am. Neurol. Assoc.* **1999**, *46*, 606–611. [CrossRef]
51. Gervil, M. The relative role of genetic and environmental factors in migraine without aura. *Am. Acad. Neurol.* **1999**, *53*, 995. [CrossRef] [PubMed]
52. Russell, M.B. Genetics of migraine without aura, migraine with aura, migrainous disorder, head trauma migraine without aura and tension-type headache. *Cephalalgia* **2001**, *21*, 778–780. [CrossRef] [PubMed]
53. Mulder, E.J.; Van Baal, C.; Gaist, D.; Kallela, M.; Kaprio, J.; Svensson, D.A.; Nyholt, D.R.; Martin, N.G.; Macgregor, A.J.; Cherkas, L.F.; et al. Genetic and Environmental Influences on Migraine: A Twin Study Across Six Countries. *Twin Res.* **2003**, *6*, 422–431. [CrossRef] [PubMed]
54. Polderman, T.J.C.; Benyamin, B.; De Leeuw, C.A.; Sullivan, P.F.; Van Bochoven, A.; Visscher, P.M.; Posthuma, D. Meta-analysis of the heritability of human traits based on fifty years of twin studies. *Nat. Genet.* **2015**, *47*, 702–709. [CrossRef] [PubMed]
55. Bigal, M.E.; Lipton, R.B.; Winner, P.; Reed, M.L.; Diamond, S.; Stewart, W.F. Migraine in adolescents: Association with socioeconomic status and family history. *Neurology* **2007**, *69*, 16–25. [CrossRef] [PubMed]
56. Russell, M.B.; Iselius, L.; Olesen, J. Migraine without aura and migraine with aura are inherited disorders. *Cephalalgia* **1996**, *16*, 305–309. [CrossRef] [PubMed]
57. Stewart, W.F.; Bigal, M.E.; Kolodner, K.; Dowson, A.; Liberman, J.N.; Lipton, R.B. Familial risk of migraine Variation by proband age at onset and headache severity. *Am. Acad. Neurol.* **2006**, *66*, 344–348. [CrossRef] [PubMed]
58. Russell, M.B.; Ulrich, V.; Gervil, M.; Olesen, J. Migraine Without Aura and Migraine With Aura Are Distinct Disorders. A Population-Based Twin Survey. *Headache J. Head. Face Pain* **2002**, *42*, 332–336. [CrossRef] [PubMed]
59. Devoto, M.; Lozito, A.; Staffa, G.; D'Alessandro, R.; Sacquegna, T.; Romeo, G. Segregation analysis of migraine in 128 families. *Cephalalgia* **1986**, *6*, 101–105. [CrossRef]
60. Mochi, M.; Sangiorgi, S.; Cortelli, P.; Carelli, V.; Scapoli, C.; Crisci, M.; Monari, L.; Pierangeli, G.; Montagna, P. Testing models for genetic determination of migraine. *Cephalalgia* **1993**, *13*, 389–394. [CrossRef]
61. Montagna, P. Migraine genetics. *Expert Rev. Neurother.* **2008**, *8*, 1321–1330. [CrossRef] [PubMed]
62. D'Amico, D.; Leone, M.; Macciardi, F.; Valentini, S.; Bussone, G. Genetic transmission of migraine without aura: A study of 68 families. *Ital. J. Neurol. Sci.* **1991**, *12*, 581–584. [CrossRef] [PubMed]
63. Gormley, P.; Anttila, V.; Winsvold, B.S.; Palta, P.; Esko, T.; Pers, T.H.; Farh, K.-H.; Cuenca-Leon, E.; Muona, M.; Furlotte, N.A.; et al. Meta-analysis of 375,000 individuals identifies 38 susceptibility loci for migraine. *Nat. Genet.* **2016**, *48*, 856–866. [CrossRef] [PubMed]
64. Nyholt, D.R.; Gillespie, N.G.; Heath, A.C.; Merikangas, K.R.; Duffy, D.L.; Martin, N.G. Latent class and genetic analysis does not support migraine with aura and migraine without aura as separate entities. *Genet. Epidemiol.* **2004**, *26*, 231–244. [CrossRef] [PubMed]
65. Ligthart, L.; Boomsma, D.I.; Martin, N.G.; Stubbe, J.H.; Nyholt, D.R. Migraine With Aura and Migraine Without Aura Are Not Distinct Entities: Further Evidence From a Large Dutch Population Study. *Twin Res. Hum. Genet.* **2006**, *9*, 54–63. [CrossRef] [PubMed]
66. de Vries, B.; Frants, R.R.; Ferrari, M.D.; van den Maagdenberg, A.M. Molecular genetics of migraine. *Hum. Genet.* **2009**, *126*, 115–132. [CrossRef] [PubMed]
67. Launer, L.J.; Terwindt, G.M.; Ferrari, M.D. The prevalence and characteristics of migraine in a population-based cohort: The GEM study. *Neurology* **1999**, *53*, 537. [CrossRef] [PubMed]
68. Nyholt, D.R.; Borsook, D.; Griffiths, L.R. Migrainomics—Identifying brain and genetic markers of migraine. *Nat. Rev. Neurol.* **2017**, *13*, 725–741. [CrossRef] [PubMed]
69. Gasparini, C.; Sutherland, H.; Griffiths, L. Studies on the Pathophysiology and Genetic Basis of Migraine. *Curr. Genom.* **2013**, *14*, 300–315. [CrossRef]
70. Anttila, V.; Bulik-Sullivan, B.; Finucane, H.K.; Walters, R.K.; Bras, J.; Duncan, L.; Escott-Price, V.; Falcone, G.J.; Gormley, P.; Malik, R.; et al. Analysis of shared heritability in common disorders of the brain. *Science* **2018**, *360*, eaap8757. [CrossRef]
71. Nyholt, D.R.; Anttila, V.; Winsvold, B.S.; Kurth, T.; Stefansson, H.; Kallela, M.; Malik, R.; Vries, B.D.; Terwindt, G.M.; Ikram, M.A.; et al. Concordance of genetic risk across migraine subgroups: Impact on current and future genetic association studies. *Cephalalgia* **2015**, *35*, 489–499. [CrossRef]
72. Zhao, H.; Eising, E.; De Vries, B.; Vijfhuizen, L.S.; Anttila, V.; Winsvold, B.S.; Kurth, T.; Stefansson, H.; Kallela, M.; Malik, R.; et al. Gene-based pleiotropy across migraine with aura and migraine without aura patient groups. *Cephalalgia* **2016**, *36*, 648–657. [CrossRef] [PubMed]

73. Freilinger, T.; Anttila, V.; De Vries, B.; Malik, R.; Kallela, M.; Terwindt, G.M.; Pozo-Rosich, P.; Winsvold, B.; Nyholt, D.R.; Van Oosterhout, W.P.J.; et al. Genome-wide association analysis identifies susceptibility loci for migraine without aura. *Nat. Genet.* **2012**, *44*, 777–782. [CrossRef]
74. Dias, A.; Mariz, T.; Sousa, A.; Lemos, C.; Alves-Ferreira, M. A review of migraine genetics: Gathering genomic and transcriptomic factors. *Hum. Genet.* **2022**, *141*, 1–14. [CrossRef]
75. Sepulveda-Sanchez, J.; Matia-Frances, R.; Martinez-Salio, A.; González-de la Aleja-Tejera, J.; Porta-Etessam, J. Homocysteine and cerebrovascular disease. *Rev. Neurol.* **2004**, *38*, 347–358. [PubMed]
76. Rozen, R. Genetic predisposition to hyperhomocysteinemia: Deficiency of methylenetetrahydrofolate reductase (MTHFR). *Thromb. Haemost.* **1997**, *78*, 523–526. [CrossRef] [PubMed]
77. Todt, U.; Freudenberg, J.; Goebel, I.; Netzer, C.; Heinze, A.; Heinze-Kuhn, K.; Göbel, H.; Kubisch, C. MTHFR C677T polymorphism and migraine with aura. *Ann. Neurol.* **2006**, *60*, 621–622. [CrossRef]
78. De Vries, B.; Anttila, V.; Freilinger, T.; Wessman, M.; Kaunisto, M.A.; Kallela, M.; Artto, V.; Vijfhuizen, L.S.; Göbel, H.; Dichgans, M.; et al. Systematic re-evaluation of genes from candidate gene association studies in migraine using a large genome-wide association data set. *Cephalalgia* **2016**, *36*, 604–614. [CrossRef]
79. Akerman, S.; Goadsby, P. Dopamine and migraine: Biology and clinical implications. *Cephalalgia* **2007**, *27*, 1308–1314. [CrossRef]
80. Chen, J.; Qin, Z.; Szele, F.; Bai, G.; Weiss, B. Neuronal localization and modulation of the D2 dopamine receptor mRNA in brain of normal mice and mice lesioned with 6-hydroxydopamine. *Neuropharmacology* **1991**, *30*, 927–941. [CrossRef]
81. Lazarov, N.; Pilgrim, C. Localization of D1 and D2 dopamine receptors in the rat mesencephalic trigeminal nucleus by immunocytochemistry and in situ hybridization. *Neurosci. Lett.* **1997**, *236*, 83–86. [CrossRef] [PubMed]
82. Peterfreund, R.A.; Kosofsky, B.E.; Fink, J.S. Cellular localization of dopamine D2 receptor messenger RNA in the rat trigeminal ganglion. *Anesth. Analg.* **1995**, *81*, 1181–1185.
83. Bes, A.; Dupui, P.; Güell, A.; Bessoles, G.; Geraud, G. Pharmacological exploration of dopamine hypersensitivity in migraine patients. *Int. J. Clin. Pharmacol. Res.* **1986**, *6*, 189–192. [PubMed]
84. Piccini, P.; Pavese, N.; Palombo, C.; Pittella, G.; Distante, A.; Bonuccelli, U. Transcranial Doppler ultrasound in migraine and tension-type headache after apomorphine administration: Double-blind crossover versus placebo study. *Cephalalgia* **1995**, *15*, 399–403. [CrossRef] [PubMed]
85. Edvinsson, L.; Hardebo, J.; McCulloch, J.; Owman, C. Effects of dopaminergic agonists and antagonists on isolated cerebral blood vessels. *Acta Physiol. Scand.* **1978**, *104*, 349–359. [CrossRef] [PubMed]
86. Erdal, M.E.; Herken, H.; Yilmaz, M.; Bayazit, Y.A. Significance of the catechol-O-methyltransferase gene polymorphism in migraine. *Mol. Brain Res.* **2001**, *94*, 193–196. [CrossRef]
87. Gürsoy, S.; Erdal, E.; Herken, H.; Madenci, E.; Alaşehirli, B.; Erdal, N. Significance of catechol-O-methyltransferase gene polymorphism in fibromyalgia syndrome. *Rheumatol. Int.* **2003**, *23*, 104–107. [CrossRef] [PubMed]
88. Hagen, K.; Pettersen, E.; Stovner, L.J.; Skorpen, F.; Zwart, J.-A. The association between headache and Val158Met polymorphism in the catechol-O-methyltransferase gene: The HUNT Study. *J. Headache Pain* **2006**, *7*, 70–74. [CrossRef] [PubMed]
89. Fernandez, F.; Colson, N.; Quinlan, S.; MacMillan, J.; Lea, R.; Griffiths, L. Association between migraine and a functional polymorphism at the dopamine β-hydroxylase locus. *Neurogenetics* **2009**, *10*, 199–208. [CrossRef]
90. Nyholt, D.R.; LaForge, K.S.; Kallela, M.; Alakurtti, K.; Anttila, V.; Farkkila, M.; Hamalainen, E.; Kaprio, J.; Kaunisto, M.A.; Heath, A.C.; et al. A high-density association screen of 155 ion transport genes for involvement with common migraine. *Hum. Mol. Genet.* **2008**, *17*, 3318–3331. [CrossRef]
91. Curtain, R.; Tajouri, L.; Lea, R.; MacMillan, J.; Griffiths, L. No mutations detected in the INSR gene in a chromosome 19p13 linked migraine pedigree. *Eur. J. Med. Genet.* **2006**, *49*, 57–62. [CrossRef]
92. McCarthy, L.C.; Hosford, D.A.; Riley, J.H.; Bird, M.I.; White, N.J.; Hewett, D.R.; Peroutka, S.J.; Griffiths, L.R.; Boyd, P.R.; Lea, R.A.; et al. Single-nucleotide polymorphism alleles in the insulin receptor gene are associated with typical migraine. *Genomics* **2001**, *78*, 135–149. [CrossRef]
93. Curtain, R.; Lea, R.A.; Quinlan, S.; Bellis, C.; Tajouri, L.; Hughes, R.; Macmillan, J.; Griffiths, L.R. Investigation of the low-density lipoprotein receptor gene and cholesterol as a risk factor for migraine. *J. Neurol. Sci.* **2004**, *227*, 95–100. [CrossRef]
94. Mochi, M.; Cevoli, S.; Cortelli, P.; Pierangeli, G.; Scapoli, C.; Soriani, S.; Montagna, P. Investigation of an LDLR gene polymorphism (19p13.2) in susceptibility to migraine without aura. *J. Neurol. Sci.* **2003**, *213*, 7–10. [CrossRef] [PubMed]
95. Russo, L.; Mariotti, P.; Sangiorgi, E.; Giordano, T.; Ricci, I.; Lupi, F.; Chiera, R.; Guzzetta, F.; Neri, G.; Gurrieri, F. A New Susceptibility Locus for Migraine with Aura in the 15q11-q13 Genomic Region Containing Three GABA-A Receptor Genes. *Am. J. Hum. Genet.* **2005**, *76*, 327–333. [CrossRef]
96. Carlsson, A.; Forsgren, L.; Nylander, P.-O.; Hellman, U.; Forsman-Semb, K.; Holmgren, G.; Holmberg, D.; Holmberg, M. Identification of a susceptibility locus for migraine with and without aura on 6p12.2-p21.1. *Neurology* **2002**, *59*, 1804–1807. [CrossRef]
97. Wessman, M.; Kallela, M.; Kaunisto, M.A.; Marttila, P.; Sobel, E.; Hartiala, J.; Oswell, G.; Leal, S.M.; Papp, J.C.; Hämäläinen, E.; et al. A Susceptibility Locus for Migraine with Aura, on Chromosome 4q24. *Am. J. Hum. Genet.* **2002**, *70*, 652–662. [CrossRef] [PubMed]

98. Björnsson, Á.; Gudmundsson, G.; Gudfinnsson, E.; Hrafnsdóttir, M.; Benedikz, J.; Skúladóttir, S.; Kristjánsson, K.; Frigge, M.L.; Kong, A.; Stefánsson, K.; et al. Localization of a Gene for Migraine without Aura to Chromosome 4q21. *Am. J. Hum. Genet.* **2003**, *73*, 986–993. [CrossRef] [PubMed]
99. Jones, K.W.; Ehm, M.G.; Pericak-Vance, M.A.; Haines, J.L.; Boyd, P.R.; Peroutka, S.J. Migraine with aura susceptibility locus on chromosome 19p13 is distinct from the familial hemiplegic migraine locus. *Genomics* **2001**, *78*, 150–154. [CrossRef]
100. Lea, R.A.; Shepherd, G.A.; Curtain, R.P.; Nyholt, D.R.; Quinlan, S.; Brimage, P.J.; Griffiths, L.R. A typical migraine susceptibility region localizes to chromosome 1q31. *Neurogenetics* **2002**, *4*, 17–22. [CrossRef]
101. Cader, Z.M.; Noble-Topham, S.; Dyment, D.A.; Cherny, S.S.; Brown, J.D.; Rice, G.P.; Ebers, G.C. Significant linkage to migraine with aura on chromosome 11q24. *Hum. Mol. Genet.* **2003**, *12*, 2511–2517. [CrossRef] [PubMed]
102. Soragna, D.; Vettori, A.; Carraro, G.; Marchioni, E.; Vazza, G.; Bellini, S.; Tupler, R.; Savoldi, F.; Mostacciuolo, M. A locus for migraine without aura maps on chromosome 14q21.2-q22.3. *Am. J. Hum. Genet.* **2003**, *72*, 161–167. [CrossRef] [PubMed]
103. Anttila, V.; Nyholt, D.R.; Kallela, M.; Artto, V.; Vepsäläinen, S.; Jakkula, E.; Wennerström, A.; Tikka-Kleemola, P.; Kaunisto, M.A.; Hämäläinen, E.; et al. Consistently Replicating Locus Linked to Migraine on 10q22-q23. *Am. J. Hum. Genet.* **2008**, *82*, 1051–1063. [CrossRef] [PubMed]
104. Ligthart, L.; Nyholt, D.R.; Hottenga, J.-J.; Distel, M.A.; Willemsen, G.; Boomsma, D.I. A genome-wide linkage scan provides evidence for both new and previously reported loci influencing common migraine. *Am. J. Med. Genet. Part. B Neuropsychiatr. Genet.* **2008**, *147B*, 1186–1195. [CrossRef] [PubMed]
105. Aulchenko, Y.S.; Hoppenbrouwers, I.A.; Ramagopalan, S.V.; Broer, L.; Jafari, N.; Hillert, J.; Link, J.; Lundström, W.; Greiner, E.; Dessa Sadovnick, A. Genetic variation in the KIF1B locus influences susceptibility to multiple sclerosis. *Nat. Genet.* **2008**, *40*, 1402–1403. [CrossRef]
106. Hindorff, L.A.; Sethupathy, P.; Junkins, H.A.; Ramos, E.M.; Mehta, J.P.; Collins, F.S.; Manolio, T.A. Potential etiologic and functional implications of genome-wide association loci for human diseases and traits. *Proc. Natl. Acad. Sci. USA* **2009**, *106*, 9362–9367. [CrossRef] [PubMed]
107. Anttila, V.; Winsvold, B.S.; Gormley, P.; Kurth, T.; Bettella, F.; McMahon, G.; Kallela, M.; Malik, R.; De Vries, B.; Terwindt, G.; et al. Genome-wide meta-analysis identifies new susceptibility loci for migraine. *Nat. Genet.* **2013**, *45*, 912–917. [CrossRef] [PubMed]
108. Chasman, D.I.; Schürks, M.; Anttila, V.; De Vries, B.; Schminke, U.; Launer, L.J.; Terwindt, G.M.; Van Den Maagdenberg, A.M.J.M.; Fendrich, K.; Völzke, H.; et al. Genome-wide association study reveals three susceptibility loci for common migraine in the general population. *Nat. Genet.* **2011**, *43*, 695–698. [CrossRef] [PubMed]
109. Gupta, R.M.; Hadaya, J.; Trehan, A.; Zekavat, S.M.; Roselli, C.; Klarin, D.; Emdin, C.A.; Hilvering, C.R.; Bianchi, V.; Mueller, C.; et al. A genetic variant associated with five vascular diseases is a distal regulator of endothelin-1 gene expression. *Cell* **2017**, *170*, 522–533.e515. [CrossRef]
110. Guo, Y.; Rist, P.M.; Daghlas, I.; Giulianini, F.; Kurth, T.; Chasman, D.I. A genome-wide cross-phenotype meta-analysis of the association of blood pressure with migraine. *Nat. Commun.* **2020**, *11*, 3368. [CrossRef]
111. Gerring, Z.F.; Powell, J.E.; Montgomery, G.W.; Nyholt, D.R. Genome-wide analysis of blood gene expression in migraine implicates immune-inflammatory pathways. *Cephalalgia* **2018**, *38*, 292–303. [CrossRef] [PubMed]
112. Hautakangas, H.; Winsvold, B.S.; Ruotsalainen, S.E.; Bjornsdottir, G.; Harder, A.V.; Kogelman, L.J.; Thomas, L.F.; Noordam, R.; Benner, C.; Gormley, P. Genome-wide analysis of 102,084 migraine cases identifies 123 risk loci and subtype-specific risk alleles. *MedRxiv* **2021**, *54*, 152–160. [CrossRef] [PubMed]
113. Kang, D.-c.; Su, Z.-z.; Sarkar, D.; Emdad, L.; Volsky, D.J.; Fisher, P.B. Cloning and characterization of HIV-1-inducible astrocyte elevated gene-1, AEG-1. *Gene* **2005**, *353*, 8–15. [CrossRef] [PubMed]
114. Noch, E.; Khalili, K. Molecular mechanisms of necrosis in glioblastoma: The role of glutamate excitotoxicity. *Cancer Biol. Ther.* **2009**, *8*, 1791–1797. [CrossRef]
115. Iljazi, A.; Ayata, C.; Ashina, M.; Hougaard, A. The role of endothelin in the pathophysiology of migraine—A systematic review. *Curr. Pain Headache Rep.* **2018**, *22*, 27. [CrossRef] [PubMed]
116. Ishibashi, J.; Seale, P. Functions of Prdm16 in thermogenic fat cells. *Temperature* **2015**, *2*, 65–72. [CrossRef] [PubMed]
117. Thimraj, T.A.; George, L.; Asrafuzzaman, S.; Upadhyay, S.; Ganguly, K. Oxidative signaling in chronic obstructive airway diseases. In *Immunity and Inflammation in Health and Disease*; Elsevier: Amsterdam, The Netherlands, 2018; pp. 79–98.
118. Wong-Spracklen, V.M.; Kolesnik, A.; Eck, J.; Sabanathan, S.; Spasic-Boskovic, O.; Maw, A.; Baker, K. Biallelic CACNA1A variants: Review of literature and report of a child with drug-resistant epilepsy and developmental delay. *Am. J. Med. Genet. Part. A* **2022**, *188*, 3306–3311. [CrossRef]
119. Pellecchia, S.; Sepe, R.; Federico, A.; Cuomo, M.; Credendino, S.C.; Pisapia, P.; Bellevicine, C.; Nicolau-Neto, P.; Severo Ramundo, M.; Crescenzi, E. The metallophosphoesterase-domain-containing protein 2 (MPPED2) gene acts as tumor suppressor in breast cancer. *Cancers* **2019**, *11*, 797. [CrossRef]
120. Titus, A.; Marappa-Ganeshan, R. Physiology, Endothelin. In *StatPearls*; StatPearls Publishing: Treasure Island, FL, USA, 2023.
121. Wang, Z.; Gerstein, M.; Snyder, M. RNA-Seq: A revolutionary tool for transcriptomics. *Nat. Rev. Genet.* **2009**, *10*, 57–63. [CrossRef]
122. Renthal, W. Localization of migraine susceptibility genes in human brain by single-cell RNA sequencing. *Cephalalgia* **2018**, *38*, 1976–1983. [CrossRef]
123. Starobova, H.; Himaya, S.W.A.; Lewis, R.J.; Vetter, I. Transcriptomics in pain research: Insights from new and old technologies. *Mol. Omics* **2018**, *14*, 389–404. [CrossRef] [PubMed]

124. Jeong, H.; Moye, L.S.; Southey, B.R.; Hernandez, A.G.; Dripps, I.; Romanova, E.V.; Rubakhin, S.S.; Sweedler, J.V.; Pradhan, A.A.; Rodriguez-Zas, S.L. Gene network dysregulation in the trigeminal ganglia and nucleus accumbens of a model of chronic migraine-associated hyperalgesia. *Front. Syst. Neurosci.* **2018**, *12*, 63. [CrossRef] [PubMed]
125. Kogelman, L.J.; Falkenberg, K.; Halldorsson, G.H.; Poulsen, L.U.; Worm, J.; Ingason, A.; Stefansson, H.; Stefansson, K.; Hansen, T.F.; Olesen, J. Comparing migraine with and without aura to healthy controls using RNA sequencing. *Cephalalgia* **2019**, *39*, 1435–1444. [CrossRef] [PubMed]
126. Vgontzas, A.; Renthal, W. Migraine-associated gene expression in cell types of the central and peripheral nervous system. *Cephalalgia* **2020**, *40*, 517–523. [CrossRef] [PubMed]
127. Kogelman, L.J.; Falkenberg, K.; Buil, A.; Erola, P.; Courraud, J.; Laursen, S.S.; Michoel, T.; Olesen, J.; Hansen, T.F. Changes in the gene expression profile during spontaneous migraine attacks. *Sci. Rep.* **2021**, *11*, 8294. [CrossRef] [PubMed]
128. Ibrahim, O.; Sutherland, H.G.; Maksemous, N.; Smith, R.; Haupt, L.M.; Griffiths, L.R. Exploring neuronal vulnerability to head trauma using a whole exome approach. *J. Neurotrauma* **2020**, *37*, 1870–1879. [CrossRef] [PubMed]
129. Rasmussen, A.H.; Olofsson, I.; Chalmer, M.A.; Olesen, J.; Hansen, T.F. Higher burden of rare frameshift indels in genes related to synaptic transmission separate familial hemiplegic migraine from common types of migraine. *J. Med. Genet.* **2020**, *57*, 610–616. [CrossRef] [PubMed]
130. Rasmussen, A.H.; Kogelman, L.J.; Kristensen, D.M.; Chalmer, M.A.; Olesen, J.; Hansen, T.F. Functional gene networks reveal distinct mechanisms segregating in migraine families. *Brain* **2020**, *143*, 2945–2956. [CrossRef] [PubMed]
131. Rudkjobing, L.A.; Esserlind, A.-L.; Olesen, J. Future possibilities in migraine genetics. *J. Headache Pain* **2012**, *13*, 505–511. [CrossRef]
132. Vaz-Drago, R.; Custódio, N.; Carmo-Fonseca, M. Deep intronic mutations and human disease. *Hum. Genet.* **2017**, *136*, 1093–1111. [CrossRef]
133. Royal, P.; Andres-Bilbe, A.; Prado, P.Á.; Verkest, C.; Wdziekonski, B.; Schaub, S.; Baron, A.; Lesage, F.; Gasull, X.; Levitz, J.; et al. Migraine-associated TRESK mutations increase neuronal excitability through alternative translation initiation and inhibition of TREK. *Neuron* **2019**, *101*, 232–245.e236. [CrossRef] [PubMed]
134. Gazerani, P. Current evidence on potential uses of MicroRNA biomarkers for migraine: From diagnosis to treatment. *Mol. Diagn. Ther.* **2019**, *23*, 681–694. [CrossRef] [PubMed]
135. Tafuri, E.; Santovito, D.; de Nardis, V.; Marcantonio, P.; Paganelli, C.; Affaitati, G.; Bucci, M.; Mezzetti, A.; Giamberardino, M.A.; Cipollone, F. MicroRNA profiling in migraine without aura: Pilot study. *Ann. Med.* **2015**, *47*, 468–473. [CrossRef] [PubMed]
136. Joutel, A.; Vahedi, K.; Corpechot, C.; Troesch, A.; Chabriat, H.; Vayssière, C.; Cruaud, C.; Maciazek, J.; Weissenbach, J.; Bousser, M.-G.; et al. Strong clustering and stereotyped nature of Notch3 mutations in CADASIL patients. *Lancet* **1997**, *350*, 1511–1515. [CrossRef] [PubMed]
137. Tan, R.Y.Y.; Markus, H.S. CADASIL: Migraine, encephalopathy, stroke and their inter-relationships. *PLoS ONE* **2016**, *11*, e0157613. [CrossRef]
138. Liem, M.K.; Oberstein, S.A.L.; van der Grond, J.; Ferrari, M.D.; Haan, J. CADASIL and migraine: A narrative review. *Cephalalgia* **2010**, *30*, 1284–1289. [CrossRef] [PubMed]
139. Piper, R.D.; Lambert, G.A.; Duckworth, J.W. Cortical blood flow changes during spreading depression in cats. *Am. J. Physiol.-Heart Circ. Physiol.* **1991**, *261*, H96–H102. [CrossRef]
140. Tfelt-Hansen, P.; Thorbjørn Jensen, L.; Olesen, J. Delayed hyperperfusion following migraine with a prolonged aphasic aura in a patient with CADASIL. *Cephalalgia* **2008**, *28*, 899–902. [CrossRef] [PubMed]
141. Eikermann-Haerter, K.; Wang, Y.; Dilekoz, E.; Arboleda-Velasquez, J.; Artavanis-Tsakonas, S.; Joutel, A.; Moskowitz, M.; Ayata, C. Increased Susceptibility to Cortical Spreading Depression in CADASIL Mutant Mice. 2009. Available online: https://www.ncbi.nlm.nih.gov/pmc/articles/PMC3058390/ (accessed on 29 April 2024).
142. Kors, E.E.; Vanmolkot, K.R.; Haan, J.; Frants, R.R.; van den Maagdenberg, A.M.; Ferrari, M.D. Recent findings in headache genetics. *Curr. Opin. Neurol.* **2004**, *17*, 283–288. [CrossRef]
143. Romero, J.M.; Rojas-Serrano, L.F. Current Evaluation of Intracerebral Hemorrhage. *Radiol. Clin.* **2023**, *61*, 479–490. [CrossRef]
144. Itoh, Y.; Yamada, M.; Hayakawa, M.; Otomo, E.; Miyatake, T. Cerebral amyloid angiopathy: A significant cause of cerebellar as well as lobar cerebral hemorrhage in the elderly. *J. Neurol. Sci.* **1993**, *116*, 135–141. [CrossRef] [PubMed]
145. Koemans, E.A.; Voigt, S.; Rasing, I.; van Etten, E.S.; van Zwet, E.W.; van Walderveen, M.A.; Wermer, M.J.; Terwindt, G.M. Migraine with aura as early disease marker in hereditary Dutch-type cerebral amyloid angiopathy. *Stroke* **2020**, *51*, 1094–1099. [CrossRef] [PubMed]
146. Agostoni, E.; Rigamonti, A. Migraine and small vessel diseases. *Neurol. Sci.* **2012**, *33*, 51–54. [CrossRef] [PubMed]
147. Plaisier, E.; Ronco, P. COL4A1-Related Disorders. In *GeneReviews®[Internet]*; 2009 Jun 25 [updated 2016 Jul 7]; Adam, M.P., Feldman, J., Mirzaa, G.M., Pagon, R.A., Wallace, S.E., Bean, L.J.H., Gripp, K.W., Amemiya, A., Eds.; University of Washington: Seattle, WA, USA, 1993–2024. [PubMed]
148. Gould, D.B.; Phalan, F.C.; Van Mil, S.E.; Sundberg, J.P.; Vahedi, K.; Massin, P.; Bousser, M.G.; Heutink, P.; Miner, J.H.; Tournier-Lasserve, E.; et al. Role of COL4A1 in small-vessel disease and hemorrhagic stroke. *N. Engl. J. Med.* **2006**, *354*, 1489–1496. [CrossRef] [PubMed]
149. Lanfranconi, S.; Markus, H.S. COL4A1 mutations as a monogenic cause of cerebral small vessel disease: A systematic review. *Stroke* **2010**, *41*, e513–e518. [CrossRef] [PubMed]

150. Xu, Y.; Padiath, Q.S.; Shapiro, R.E.; Jones, C.R.; Wu, S.C.; Saigoh, N.; Saigoh, K.; Ptáček, L.J.; Fu, Y.-H. Functional consequences of a CKIδ mutation causing familial advanced sleep phase syndrome. *Nature* **2005**, *434*, 640–644. [CrossRef] [PubMed]
151. Cheong, J.K.; Virshup, D.M. Casein kinase 1: Complexity in the family. *Int. J. Biochem. Cell Biol.* **2011**, *43*, 465–469. [CrossRef] [PubMed]
152. Knippschild, U.; Gocht, A.; Wolff, S.; Huber, N.; Löhler, J.; Stöter, M. The casein kinase 1 family: Participation in multiple cellular processes in eukaryotes. *Cell. Signal.* **2005**, *17*, 675–689. [CrossRef]
153. Toh, K.L.; Jones, C.R.; He, Y.; Eide, E.J.; Hinz, W.A.; Virshup, D.M.; Ptácek, L.J.; Fu, Y.-H. An h Per2 phosphorylation site mutation in familial advanced sleep phase syndrome. *Science* **2001**, *291*, 1040–1043. [CrossRef]
154. Lee, H.; Chen, R.; Lee, Y.; Yoo, S.; Lee, C. Essential roles of CKIδ and CKIε in the mammalian circadian clock. *Proc. Natl. Acad. Sci. USA* **2009**, *106*, 21359–21364. [CrossRef]
155. Brennan, K.; Bates, E.A.; Shapiro, R.E.; Zyuzin, J.; Hallows, W.C.; Huang, Y.; Lee, H.-Y.; Jones, C.R.; Fu, Y.-H.; Charles, A.C.; et al. Casein kinase iδ mutations in familial migraine and advanced sleep phase. *Sci. Transl. Med.* **2013**, *5*, ra156–ra183. [CrossRef] [PubMed]
156. Lafrenière, R.G.; Rouleau, G.A. Migraine: Role of the TRESK two-pore potassium channel. *Int. J. Biochem. Cell Biol.* **2011**, *43*, 1533–1536. [CrossRef] [PubMed]
157. Kowalska, M.; Prendecki, M.; Kapelusiak-Pielok, M.; Grzelak, T.; Łagan-Jędrzejczyk, U.; Wiszniewska, M.; Kozubski, W.; Dorszewska, J. Analysis of Genetic Variants in SCN1A, SCN2A, KCNK18, TRPA1 and STX1A as a Possible Marker of Migraine. *Curr. Genom.* **2020**, *21*, 224–236. [CrossRef] [PubMed]
158. Jen, J.; Cohen, A.; Yue, Q.; Stout, J.; Vinters, H.; Nelson, S.; Baloh, R. Hereditary endotheliopathy with retinopathy, nephropathy, and stroke (HERNS). *Neurology* **1997**, *49*, 1322–1330. [CrossRef] [PubMed]
159. Elliott, D. Migraine and stroke: Current perspectives. *Neurol. Res.* **2008**, *30*, 801–812. [CrossRef] [PubMed]
160. Salloway, S.; Cummings, J. Subcortical disease and neuropsychiatric illness. *J. Neuropsychiatry Clin. Neurosci.* **1994**, *6*, 93–99. [PubMed]
161. Hirano, M.; Pavlakis, S.G. Topical review: Mitochondrial myopathy, encephalopathy, lactic acidosis, and strokelike episodes (MELAS): Current concepts. *J. Child. Neurol.* **1994**, *9*, 4–13. [CrossRef] [PubMed]
162. Hirano, M.; Ricci, E.; Koenigsberger, M.R.; Defendini, R.; Pavlakis, S.G.; DeVivo, D.C.; DiMauro, S.; Rowland, L.P. MELAS: An original case and clinical criteria for diagnosis. *Neuromuscul. Disord.* **1992**, *2*, 125–135. [CrossRef] [PubMed]
163. Ohno, K.; Isotani, E.; Hirakawa, K. MELAS presenting as migraine complicated by stroke: Case report. *Neuroradiology* **1997**, *39*, 781–784. [CrossRef] [PubMed]
164. Sproule, D.M.; Kaufmann, P. Mitochondrial encephalopathy, lactic acidosis, and strokelike episodes: Basic concepts, clinical phenotype, and therapeutic management of MELAS syndrome. *Ann. N. Y. Acad. Sci.* **2008**, *1142*, 133–158. [CrossRef]
165. Montagna, P.; Gallassi, R.; Medori, R.; Govoni, E.; Zeviani, M.; Di Mauro, S.; Lugaresi, E.; Andermann, F. MELAS syndrome: Characteristic migrainous and epileptic features and maternal transmission. *Neurology* **1988**, *38*, 751. [CrossRef] [PubMed]
166. Nakagawa, M.; Osame, M. Clinical aspects of mitochondrial encephalomyopathy—Abnormality of mitochondrial respiratory chain. *No Shinkei Brain Nerve* **1990**, *42*, 719–733. [PubMed]
167. Wong, L.J.C. Pathogenic mitochondrial DNA mutations in protein-coding genes. *Muscle Nerve Off. J. Am. Assoc. Electrodiagn. Med.* **2007**, *36*, 279–293. [CrossRef] [PubMed]
168. Buzzi, M.G.; Di Gennaro, G.; D'Onofrio, M.; Ciccarelli, O.; Santorelli, F.; Fortini, D.; Nappi, G.; Nicoletti, F.; Casali, C. mtDNA A3243G MELAS mutation is not associated with multigenerational female migraine. *Neurology* **2000**, *54*, 1005–1007. [CrossRef] [PubMed]
169. Cevoli, S.; Pallotti, F.; Morgia, C.L.; Valentino, M.L.; Pierangeli, G.; Cortelli, P.; Baruzzi, A.; Montagna, P.; Carelli, V. High frequency of migraine-only patients negative for the 3243 A>G tRNALeu mtDNA mutation in two MELAS families. *Cephalalgia* **2010**, *30*, 919–927. [CrossRef] [PubMed]
170. Wilms, A.; de Boer, I.; Terwindt, G. Retinal Vasculopathy with Cerebral Leukoencephalopathy and Systemic manifestations (RVCL-S): An update on basic science and clinical perspectives. *Cereb. Circ. Cogn. Behav.* **2022**, *3*, 100046. [CrossRef] [PubMed]
171. Ford, A.L.; Chin, V.W.; Fellah, S.; Binkley, M.M.; Bodin, A.M.; Balasetti, V.; Taiwo, Y.; Kang, P.; Lin, D.; Jen, J.C. Lesion evolution and neurodegeneration in RVCL-S: A monogenic microvasculopathy. *Neurology* **2020**, *95*, e1918–e1931. [CrossRef] [PubMed]
172. Stam, A.H.; Kothari, P.H.; Shaikh, A.; Gschwendter, A.; Jen, J.C.; Hodgkinson, S.; Hardy, T.A.; Hayes, M.; Kempster, P.A.; Kotschet, K.E.; et al. Retinal vasculopathy with cerebral leukoencephalopathy and systemic manifestations. *Brain* **2016**, *139*, 2909–2922. [CrossRef]
173. Mateen, F.; Krecke, K.; Younge, B.; Ford, A.; Shaikh, A.; Kothari, P.; Atkinson, J. Evolution of a tumor-like lesion in cerebroretinal vasculopathy and TREX1 mutation. *Neurology* **2010**, *75*, 1211–1213. [CrossRef]
174. DiFrancesco, J.C.; Novara, F.; Zuffardi, O.; Forlino, A.; Gioia, R.; Cossu, F.; Bolognesi, M.; Andreoni, S.; Saracchi, E.; Frigeni, B.; et al. TREX1 C-terminal frameshift mutations in the systemic variant of retinal vasculopathy with cerebral leukodystrophy. *Neurol. Sci.* **2015**, *36*, 323–330. [CrossRef]
175. Pelzer, N.; Hoogeveen, E.; Haan, J.; Bunnik, R.; Poot, C.; van Zwet, E.; Inderson, A.; Fogteloo, A.; Reinders, M.; Middelkoop, H.; et al. Systemic features of retinal vasculopathy with cerebral leukoencephalopathy and systemic manifestations: A monogenic small vessel disease. *J. Intern. Med.* **2019**, *285*, 317–332. [CrossRef]

176. Simard, J.M.; Francisco, G.-B.; Ballinger, W.E., Jr.; Mickle, J.P.; Quisling, R.G. Cavernous angioma: A review of 126 collected and 12 new clinical cases. *Neurosurgery* **1986**, *18*, 162–172. [CrossRef] [PubMed]
177. Requena, I.; Arias, M.; Lopez-Ibor, L.; Pereiro, I.; Barba, A.; Alonso, A.; Monton, E. Cavernomas of the central nervous system: Clinical and neuroimaging manifestations in 47 patients. *J. Neurol. Neurosurg. Psychiatry* **1991**, *54*, 590–594. [CrossRef] [PubMed]
178. Chen, D.-H.; Lipe, H.P.; Qin, Z.; Bird, T.D. Cerebral cavernous malformation: Novel mutation in a Chinese family and evidence for heterogeneity. *J. Neurol. Sci.* **2002**, *196*, 91–96. [CrossRef] [PubMed]
179. Lehnhardt, F.-G.; von Smekal, U.; Rückriem, B.; Stenzel, W.; Neveling, M.; Heiss, W.-D.; Jacobs, A.H. Value of gradient-echo magnetic resonance imaging in the diagnosis of familial cerebral cavernous malformation. *Arch. Neurol.* **2005**, *62*, 653–658. [CrossRef] [PubMed]
180. Thomsen, L.L.; Eriksen, M.K.; Romer, S.F.; Andersen, I.; Ostergaard, E.; Keiding, N.; Olesen, J.; Russell, M. An epidemiological survey of hemiplegic migraine. *Cephalalgia* **2002**, *22*, 361–375. [CrossRef] [PubMed]
181. Pietrobon, D. Familial hemiplegic migraine. *Neurotherapeutics* **2007**, *4*, 274–284. [CrossRef] [PubMed]
182. Joutel, A.; Ducros, A.; Vahedi, K.; Labauge, P.; Delrieu, O.; Pinsard, N.; Mancini, J.; Ponsot, G.; Gouttiere, F.; Gastaut, J. Genetic heterogeneity of familial hemiplegic migraine. *Am. J. Hum. Genet.* **1994**, *55*, 1166. [PubMed]
183. Thomsen, L.; Eriksen, M.; Roemer, S.; Andersen, I.; Olesen, J.; Russell, M. A population-based study of familial hemiplegic migraine suggests revised diagnostic criteria. *Brain* **2002**, *125*, 1379–1391. [CrossRef]
184. Ducros, A.; Denier, C.; Joutel, A.; Cecillon, M.; Lescoat, C.; Vahedi, K.; Darcel, F.; Vicaut, E.; Bousser, M.-G.; Tournier-Lasserve, E. The clinical spectrum of familial hemiplegic migraine associated with mutations in a neuronal calcium channel. *New Engl. J. Med.* **2001**, *345*, 17–24. [CrossRef]
185. Ducros, A.; Joutel, A.; Cecillon, M.; Tournier-Lasserve, E.; Vahedi, K.; Bousser, M.G.; Ferreira, A.; Bernard, E.; Verier, A.; Echenne, B.; et al. Mapping of a second locus for familial hemiplegic migraine to 1q21–q23 and evidence of further heterogeneity. *Ann. Neurol. Off. J. Am. Neurol. Assoc. Child. Neurol. Soc.* **1997**, *42*, 885–890. [CrossRef] [PubMed]
186. Hansen, J.M.; Hauge, A.W.; Ashina, M.; Olesen, J. Trigger factors for familial hemiplegic migraine. *Cephalalgia* **2011**, *31*, 1274–1281. [CrossRef] [PubMed]
187. Chabriat, H.; Vahedi, K.; Clark, C.; Poupon, C.; Ducros, A.; Denier, C.; Le Bihan, D.; Bousser, M. Decreased hemispheric water mobility in hemiplegic migraine related to mutation of CACNA1A gene. *Neurology* **2000**, *54*, 510. [CrossRef] [PubMed]
188. Deprez, L.; Weckhuysen, S.; Peeters, K.; Deconinck, T.; Claeys, K.G.; Claes, L.R.; Suls, A.; Van Dyck, T.; Palmini, A.; Matthijs, G.; et al. Epilepsy as part of the phenotype associated with ATP1A2 mutations. *Epilepsia* **2008**, *49*, 500–508. [CrossRef] [PubMed]
189. Pietrobon, D. Function and dysfunction of synaptic calcium channels: Insights from mouse models. *Curr. Opin. Neurobiol.* **2005**, *15*, 257–265. [CrossRef] [PubMed]
190. van den Maagdenberg, A.M.; Frants, R.R. Migraine genetics: An update. *Curr. Pain Headache Rep.* **2005**, *9*, 213–220.
191. Dichgans, M.; Herzog, J.; Freilinger, T.; Wilke, M.; Auer, D. 1H-MRS alterations in the cerebellum of patients with familial hemiplegic migraine type 1. *Neurology* **2005**, *64*, 608–613. [CrossRef] [PubMed]
192. de Boer, I.; Hansen, J.M.; Terwindt, G.M. Hemiplegic migraine. *Handb. Clin. Neurol.* **2024**, *199*, 353–365. [CrossRef] [PubMed]
193. Sanchez Del Rio, M.; Cutrer, F.M. Pathophysiology of migraine aura. *Handb. Clin. Neurol.* **2023**, *198*, 71–83. [CrossRef]
194. Loonen, I.C.M.; Voskuyl, R.A.; Schenke, M.; van Heiningen, S.H.; van den Maagdenberg, A.; Tolner, E.A. Spontaneous and optogenetically induced cortical spreading depolarization in familial hemiplegic migraine type 1 mutant mice. *Neurobiol. Dis.* **2024**, *192*, 106405. [CrossRef]
195. Ayata, C.; Shimizu-Sasamata, M.; Lo, E.; Noebels, J.; Moskowitz, M. Impaired neurotransmitter release and elevated threshold for cortical spreading depression in mice with mutations in the α1A subunit of P/Q type calcium channels. *Neuroscience* **1999**, *95*, 639–645. [CrossRef] [PubMed]
196. Wakamori, M.; Yamazaki, K.; Matsunodaira, H.; Teramoto, T.; Tanaka, I.; Niidome, T.; Sawada, K.; Nishizawa, Y.; Sekiguchi, N.; Mori, E.; et al. Single tottering mutations responsible for the neuropathic phenotype of the P-type calcium channel. *J. Biol. Chem.* **1998**, *273*, 34857–34867. [CrossRef] [PubMed]
197. van den Maagdenberg, A.M.; Pietrobon, D.; Pizzorusso, T.; Kaja, S.; Broos, L.A.; Cesetti, T.; van de Ven, R.C.; Tottene, A.; van der Kaa, J.; Plomp, J.J. A Cacna1a knockin migraine mouse model with increased susceptibility to cortical spreading depression. *Neuron* **2004**, *41*, 701–710. [CrossRef] [PubMed]
198. Tottene, A.; Conti, R.; Fabbro, A.; Vecchia, D.; Shapovalova, M.; Santello, M.; van den Maagdenberg, A.M.; Ferrari, M.D.; Pie-trobon, D. Enhanced excitatory transmission at cortical synapses as the basis for facilitated spreading depression in Ca(v)2.1 knockin migraine mice. *Neuron* **2009**, *61*, 762–773. [CrossRef] [PubMed]
199. Eikermann-Haerter, K.; Diléköz, E.; Kudo, C.; Savitz, S.I.; Waeber, C.; Baum, M.J.; Ferrari, M.D.; van den Maagdenberg, A.M.; Moskowitz, M.A.; Ayata, C. Genetic and hormonal factors modulate spreading depression and transient hemiparesis in mouse models of familial hemiplegic migraine type 1. *J. Clin. Investig.* **2009**, *119*, 99–109. [CrossRef] [PubMed]
200. Eikermann-Haerter, K.; Yuzawa, I.; Qin, T.; Wang, Y.; Baek, K.; Kim, Y.R.; Hoffmann, U.; Dilekoz, E.; Waeber, C.; Ferrari, M.D. Enhanced subcortical spreading depression in familial hemiplegic migraine type 1 mutant mice. *J. Neurosci.* **2011**, *31*, 5755–5763. [CrossRef] [PubMed]
201. De Fusco, M.; Marconi, R.; Silvestri, L.; Atorino, L.; Rampoldi, L.; Morgante, L.; Ballabio, A.; Aridon, P.; Casari, G. Haploinsufficiency of ATP1A2 encoding the Na. *Nat. Genet.* **2003**, *33*, 192–196. [PubMed]

202. Blanco, G.; Mercer, R.W. Isozymes of the Na-K-ATPase: Heterogeneity in structure, diversity in function. *Am. J. Physiol. Ren. Physiol.* **1998**, *275*, F633–F650. [CrossRef] [PubMed]
203. Crambert, G.; Hasler, U.; Beggah, A.T.; Yu, C.; Modyanov, N.N.; Horisberger, J.-D.; Lelievre, L.; Geering, K.t. Transport and pharmacological properties of nine different human Na, K-ATPase isozymes. *J. Biol. Chem.* **2000**, *275*, 1976–1986. [CrossRef] [PubMed]
204. de Carvalho Aguiar, P.; Sweadner, K.J.; Penniston, J.T.; Zaremba, J.; Liu, L.; Caton, M.; Linazasoro, G.; Borg, M.; Tijssen, M.A.; Bressman, S.B. Mutations in the Na+/K+-ATPase α3 gene ATP1A3 are associated with rapid-onset dystonia parkinsonism. *Neuron* **2004**, *43*, 169–175. [CrossRef]
205. McGrail, K.; Phillips, J.; Sweadner, K. Immunofluorescent localization of three Na, K-ATPase isozymes in the rat central nervous system: Both neurons and glia can express more than one Na, K-ATPase. *J. Neurosci.* **1991**, *11*, 381–391. [CrossRef]
206. Zhang, H.; Jiang, L.; Xian, Y.; Yang, S. Familial hemiplegic migraine type 2: A case report of an adolescent with ATP1A2 mutation. *Front. Neurol.* **2024**, *15*, 1339642. [CrossRef] [PubMed]
207. Wright, S.H. Generation of resting membrane potential. *Adv. Physiol. Educ.* **2004**, *28*, 139–142. [CrossRef] [PubMed]
208. D'Ambrosio, R.; Gordon, D.S.; Winn, H.R. Differential role of KIR channel and Na+/K+-pump in the regulation of extracellular K+ in rat hippocampus. *J. Neurophysiol.* **2002**, *87*, 87–102. [CrossRef] [PubMed]
209. Ransom, C.B.; Ransom, B.R.; Sontheimer, H. Activity-dependent extracellular K+ accumulation in rat optic nerve: The role of glial and axonal Na+ pumps. *J. Physiol.* **2000**, *522*, 427–442. [CrossRef] [PubMed]
210. Anderson, C.M.; Swanson, R.A. Astrocyte glutamate transport: Review of properties, regulation, and physiological functions. *Glia* **2000**, *32*, 1–14. [CrossRef] [PubMed]
211. Rose, C.R.; Ziemens, D.; Untiet, V.; Fahlke, C. Molecular and cellular physiology of sodium-dependent glutamate transporters. *Brain Res. Bull.* **2018**, *136*, 3–16. [CrossRef]
212. Rose, E.M.; Koo, J.C.; Antflick, J.E.; Ahmed, S.M.; Angers, S.; Hampson, D.R. Glutamate transporter coupling to Na, K-ATPase. *J. Neurosci.* **2009**, *29*, 8143–8155. [CrossRef]
213. Cholet, N.; Pellerin, L.; Magistretti, P.; Hamel, E. Similar perisynaptic glial localization for the Na+, K+-ATPase α2 subunit and the glutamate transporters GLAST and GLT-1 in the rat somatosensory cortex. *Cereb. Cortex* **2002**, *12*, 515–525. [CrossRef] [PubMed]
214. Haglund, M.M.; Schwartzkroin, P.A. Role of Na-K pump potassium regulation and IPSPs in seizures and spreading depression in immature rabbit hippocampal slices. *J. Neurophysiol.* **1990**, *63*, 225–239. [CrossRef]
215. Hoefnagels, W.; Black, D.; Sandkuijl, L.; Frants, R.; Ferrari, M.; van den Maagdenberg, A. Novel mutations in the Na?, K?-ATPase pump gene ATP1A2 associated with familial hemiplegic migraine and benign familial infantile convulsions. *Ann. Neurol.* **2003**, *54*, 360Volk.
216. Spadaro, M.; Ursu, S.; Lehmann-Horn, F.; Liana, V.; Giovanni, A.; Paola, G.; Frontali, M.; Jurkat-Rott, K. A G301R Na+/K+-ATPase mutation causes familial hemiplegic migraine type 2 with cerebellar signs. *Neurogenetics* **2004**, *5*, 177–185. [CrossRef]
217. Jurkat-Rott, K.; Freilinger, T.; Dreier, J.; Herzog, J.; Göbel, H.; Petzold, G.; Montagna, P.; Gasser, T.; Lehmann-Horn, F.; Dichgans, M. Variability of familial hemiplegic migraine with novel A1A2 Na+/K+-ATPase variants. *Neurology* **2004**, *62*, 1857–1861. [CrossRef] [PubMed]
218. Riant, F.; De Fusco, M.; Aridon, P.; Ducros, A.; Ploton, C.; Marchelli, F.; Maciazek, J.; Bousser, M.G.; Casari, G.; Tournier-Lasserve, E. ATP1A2 mutations in 11 families with familial hemiplegic migraine. *Hum. Mutat.* **2005**, *26*, 281. [CrossRef] [PubMed]
219. Koenderink, J.B.; Zifarelli, G.; Qiu, L.Y.; Schwarz, W.; De Pont, J.J.H.; Bamberg, E.; Friedrich, T. Na, K-ATPase mutations in familial hemiplegic migraine lead to functional inactivation. *Biochim. Biophys. Acta (BBA)-Biomembr.* **2005**, *1669*, 61–68. [CrossRef] [PubMed]
220. Segall, L.; Mezzetti, A.; Scanzano, R.; Gargus, J.J.; Purisima, E.; Blostein, R. Alterations in the α2 isoform of Na, K-ATPase associated with familial hemiplegic migraine type 2. *Proc. Natl. Acad. Sci. USA* **2005**, *102*, 11106–11111. [CrossRef] [PubMed]
221. Vanmolkot, K.R.; Kors, E.E.; Hottenga, J.J.; Terwindt, G.M.; Haan, J.; Hoefnagels, W.A.; Black, D.F.; Sandkuijl, L.A.; Frants, R.R.; Ferrari, M.D. Novel mutations in the Na+, K+-ATPase pump gene ATP1A2 associated with familial hemiplegic migraine and benign familial infantile convulsions. *Ann. Neurol.* **2003**, *54*, 360–366. [CrossRef] [PubMed]
222. Leo, L.; Gherardini, L.; Barone, V.; De Fusco, M.; Pietrobon, D.; Pizzorusso, T.; Casari, G. Increased susceptibility to cortical spreading depression in the mouse model of familial hemiplegic migraine type 2. *PLoS Genet.* **2011**, *7*, e1002129. [CrossRef]
223. Ikeda, K.; Onaka, T.; Yamakado, M.; Nakai, J.; Ishikawa, T.-o.; Taketo, M.M.; Kawakami, K. Degeneration of the amygdala/piriform cortex and enhanced fear/anxiety behaviors in sodium pump α2 subunit (Atp1a2)-deficient mice. *J. Neurosci.* **2003**, *23*, 4667–4676. [CrossRef] [PubMed]
224. Ikeda, K.; Onimaru, H.; Yamada, J.; Inoue, K.; Ueno, S.; Onaka, T.; Toyoda, H.; Arata, A.; Ishikawa, T.-o.; Taketo, M.M. Malfunction of respiratory-related neuronal activity in Na+, K+-ATPase α2 subunit-deficient mice is attributable to abnormal Cl-homeostasis in brainstem neurons. *J. Neurosci.* **2004**, *24*, 10693–10701. [CrossRef]
225. James, P.F.; Grupp, I.L.; Grupp, G.; Woo, A.L.; Askew, G.R.; Croyle, M.L.; Walsh, R.A.; Lingrel, J.B. Identification of a specific role for the Na, K-ATPase α2 isoform as a regulator of calcium in the heart. *Mol. Cell* **1999**, *3*, 555–563. [CrossRef]
226. Li, Y.; Tang, W.; Kang, L.; Kong, S.; Dong, Z.; Zhao, D.; Liu, R.; Yu, S. Functional correlation of ATP1A2 mutations with phenotypic spectrum: From pure hemiplegic migraine to its variant forms. *J. Headache Pain* **2021**, *22*, 92. [CrossRef] [PubMed]

227. Dichgans, M.; Freilinger, T.; Eckstein, G.; Babini, E.; Lorenz-Depiereux, B.; Biskup, S.; Ferrari, M.D.; Herzog, J.; van den Maagdenberg, A.M.; Pusch, M. Mutation in the neuronal voltage-gated sodium channel SCN1A in familial hemiplegic migraine. *Lancet* **2005**, *366*, 371–377. [CrossRef]
228. Gong, B.; Rhodes, K.J.; Bekele-Arcuri, Z.; Trimmer, J.S. Type I and type II Na+ channel α-subunit polypeptides exhibit distinct spatial and temporal patterning, and association with auxiliary subunits in rat brain. *J. Comp. Neurol.* **1999**, *412*, 342–352. [CrossRef]
229. Johnston, D.; Magee, J.C.; Colbert, C.M.; Christie, B.R. Active properties of neuronal dendrites. *Annu. Rev. Neurosci.* **1996**, *19*, 165–186. [CrossRef]
230. Yu, F.H.; Mantegazza, M.; Westenbroek, R.E.; Robbins, C.A.; Kalume, F.; Burton, K.A.; Spain, W.J.; McKnight, G.S.; Scheuer, T.; Catterall, W.A. Reduced sodium current in GABAergic interneurons in a mouse model of severe myoclonic epilepsy in infancy. *Nat. Neurosci.* **2006**, *9*, 1142–1149. [CrossRef] [PubMed]
231. Gargus, J.J.; Tournay, A. Novel mutation confirms seizure locus SCN1A is also familial hemiplegic migraine locus FHM3. *Pediatr. Neurol.* **2007**, *37*, 407–410. [CrossRef]
232. Dhifallah, S.; Lancaster, E.; Merrill, S.; Leroudier, N.; Mantegazza, M.; Cestèle, S. Gain of function for the SCN1A/hNav1.1-L1670W mutation responsible for familial hemiplegic migraine. *Front. Mol. Neurosci.* **2018**, *11*, 232. [CrossRef]
233. Cestèle, S.; Schiavon, E.; Rusconi, R.; Franceschetti, S.; Mantegazza, M. Nonfunctional NaV1.1 familial hemiplegic migraine mutant transformed into gain of function by partial rescue of folding defects. *Proc. Natl. Acad. Sci. USA* **2013**, *110*, 17546–17551. [CrossRef] [PubMed]
234. Kahlig, K.M.; Rhodes, T.H.; Pusch, M.; Freilinger, T.; Pereira-Monteiro, J.M.; Ferrari, M.D.; Van Den Maagdenberg, A.M.; Dichgans, M.; George, A.L., Jr. Divergent sodium channel defects in familial hemiplegic migraine. *Proc. Natl. Acad. Sci. USA* **2008**, *105*, 9799–9804. [CrossRef]
235. Jansen, N.A.; Dehghani, A.; Linssen, M.M.; Breukel, C.; Tolner, E.A.; van den Maagdenberg, A.M. First FHM3 mouse model shows spontaneous cortical spreading depolarizations. *Ann. Clin. Transl. Neurol.* **2020**, *7*, 132–138. [CrossRef]
236. Desroches, M.; Faugeras, O.; Krupa, M.; Mantegazza, M. Modeling cortical spreading depression induced by the hyperactivity of interneurons. *J. Comput. Neurosci.* **2019**, *47*, 125–140. [CrossRef] [PubMed]
237. Wiwanitkit, V. FHM3 in familial hemiplegic migraine is more resistant to mutation than FHM1 and FHM2. *J. Neurol. Sci.* **2009**, *277*, 76–79. [CrossRef]
238. Dias, A.; Santos, M.; Carvalho, E.; Felicio, D.; Silva, P.; Alves, I.; Pinho, T.; Sousa, A.; Alves-Ferreira, M.; Lemos, C. Functional characterization of a novel PRRT2 variant found in a Portuguese patient with hemiplegic migraine. *Clin. Genet.* **2023**, *104*, 479–485. [CrossRef] [PubMed]
239. Sen, K.; Genser, I.; DiFazio, M.; DiSabella, M. Haploinsufficiency of PRRT2 Leading to Familial Hemiplegic Migraine in Chromosome 16p11.2 Deletion Syndrome. *Neuropediatrics* **2022**, *53*, 279–282. [CrossRef]
240. Nandyala, A.; Shah, T.; Ailani, J. Hemiplegic Migraine. *Curr. Neurol. Neurosci. Rep.* **2023**, *23*, 381–387. [CrossRef]
241. Suzuki-Muromoto, S.; Kosaki, R.; Kosaki, K.; Kubota, M. Familial hemiplegic migraine with a PRRT2 mutation: Phenotypic variations and carbamazepine efficacy. *Brain Dev.* **2020**, *42*, 293–297. [CrossRef]
242. Méneret, A.; Gaudebout, C.; Riant, F.; Vidailhet, M.; Depienne, C.; Roze, E. PRRT2 mutations and paroxysmal disorders. *Eur. J. Neurol.* **2013**, *20*, 872–878. [CrossRef] [PubMed]
243. Hasirci Bayir, B.R.; Tutkavul, K.; Eser, M.; Baykan, B. Epilepsy in patients with familial hemiplegic migraine. *Seizure* **2021**, *88*, 87–94. [CrossRef] [PubMed]

Disclaimer/Publisher's Note: The statements, opinions and data contained in all publications are solely those of the individual author(s) and contributor(s) and not of MDPI and/or the editor(s). MDPI and/or the editor(s) disclaim responsibility for any injury to people or property resulting from any ideas, methods, instructions or products referred to in the content.

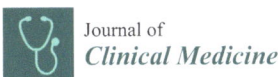

Article

Predictors of Headaches and Quality of Life in Women with Ophthalmologically Resolved Idiopathic Intracranial Hypertension

Anat Horev [1,2,†], Sapir Aharoni-Bar [3,†], Mark Katson [4], Erez Tsumi [5], Tamir Regev [5], Yair Zlotnik [1,2], Ron Biederko [6], Gal Ifergane [1,2], Ilan Shelef [2,7], Tal Eliav [8], Gal Ben-Arie [2,7,‡] and Asaf Honig [1,2,*,‡]

1. Department of Neurology, Soroka University Medical Center, Beer Sheva 8453227, Israel; anathorev@clalit.org.il (A.H.); yairzl@clalit.org.il (Y.Z.); galif@clalit.org.il (G.I.)
2. Faculty of Health Sciences, Ben Gurion University of the Negev, Beer Sheva 8453227, Israel; ilans@clalit.org.il (I.S.); galbe@clalit.org.il (G.B.-A.)
3. Ben-Gurion Medical School, Soroka University Medical Center, Beer Sheva 8453227, Israel; sapira.bc@gmail.com
4. Rambam Health Care Campus, Haifa 3109601, Israel; m_katson@rmc.gov.il
5. Department of Ophthalmology, Soroka University Medical Center, Beer Sheva 8453227, Israel; erezts@clalit.org.il (E.T.); tamirre@clalit.org.il (T.R.)
6. Clinical Research Center, Soroka University Medical Center, Beer Sheva 8453227, Israel; rbiederko@gmail.com
7. Department of Radiology, Soroka University Medical Center, Beer Sheva 8453227, Israel
8. Department of Internal Medicine, Jefferson Einstein Philadelphia Hospital, Philadelphia, PA 19141, USA; talzus@post.bgu.ac.il
* Correspondence: asaf.honig2@gmail.com
† These authors contributed equally to this work and share first authorship.
‡ These authors share last authorship.

Abstract: Background/objectives: The aim of this study was to evaluate the long-term outcomes of a cohort of ophthalmologically resolved female idiopathic intracranial hypertension (IIH) patients. **Methods:** Our cross-sectional study included adult females with at least 6 months of ophthalmologically resolved IIH. Patients with papilledema or who underwent IIH-targeted surgical intervention were excluded. Participants completed a questionnaire consisting of medical information, the Migraine Disability Assessment Scale (MIDAS) and the Headache Impact Test (HIT-6). Electronic medical records and the results of imaging upon diagnosis were retrospectively reviewed. **Results:** One-hundred-and-four participants (mean age 35.5 ± 11.9 years) were included (7.85 ± 7 years post-IIH diagnosis). Patients with moderate–severe disability according to the MIDAS scale (n = 68, 65.4%) were younger (32.4 ± 8.9 vs. 41.5 ± 14.4 year-old, $p < 0.001$), had a shorter time interval from IIH diagnosis (5.9 ± 5.3 vs. 11.7 ± 8.5 years, $p < 0.001$), and had lower FARB scores (indicating a more narrowed transverse-sigmoid junction; 1.28 ± 1.82 vs. 2.47 ± 2.3, $p = 0.02$) in comparison to patients with low–mild disability scores. In multivariate analysis, a lower FARB score (OR 1.28, 95% CI 0.89–1.75, $p = 0.12$) and younger age (OR 1.09, 95% CI 0.98–1.19, $p = 0.13$) showed a trend toward an association with a moderate–severe MIDAS score. Moreover, in the sub-analysis of patients with a moderate–severe MIDAS scale score, the 10 patients with the highest MIDAS scores had a low FARB score (1.6 ± 1.1 vs. 2.7 ± 2.4, $p = 0.041$). **Conclusions:** High numbers of patients with ophthalmologically resolved IIH continue to suffer from related symptoms. Symptoms may be associated with the length of time from the diagnosis of IIH and a lower FARB score.

Keywords: carbonic anhydrase inhibitors; headache; idiopathic intracranial hypertension; transverse sinuses; quality of life; questionnaire

1. Introduction

Idiopathic intracranial hypertension (IIH), also known as pseudotumor cerebri, is a neurological disorder characterized by elevated intracranial pressure (ICP) with no apparent cause. The underlying etiology of IIH is increased pressure in the dural venous system, but several factors may play a role in the condition's pathogenesis. IIH predominantly affects young, obese women during their childbearing years. Diagnosis is based on papilledema, normal cerebrospinal fluid analysis, and increased opening pressure on lumbar puncture with no apparent secondary cause of intracranial hypertension [1]. Symptoms may include chronic, severe headaches, transient visual obscurations, pulsatile tinnitus, cognitive dysfunction, and depression. Vision loss is the most concerning symptom as it can lead to blindness [2].

While vision loss in patients with IIH can be evaluated with neuro-ophthalmologic tests, assessing and treating headaches and other IIH-associated symptoms can be more challenging. Moreover, despite their significant impact on daily function and quality of life (QoL), these subjective symptoms are often not considered medically dangerous and so may be overlooked.

The primary goal of IIH treatment is to preserve vision and reduce headaches. Weight loss and medications, primarily carbonic anhydrase inhibitors (CAIs), are first-line treatments for IIH. However, these medications can have a wide range of side effects, with incidence rates as high as 80–100%. Furthermore, more than 10% of patients with IIH are intolerant or nonresponsive to high-dose CAI medical therapy [3–7]. In these cases, surgical procedures such as ventriculoperitoneal shunt, optic nerve fenestration, or transverse sinus stent may be considered [8].

In addition to the potential for severe visual loss and the often-debilitating related symptoms mentioned above, poor QoL has emerged as a key morbidity for patients with IIH [9]. IIH has a significant impact on patient QoL, with headaches identified as the main contributor to reduced QoL. However, treatment with the goal of improving QoL can be difficult, especially in patients who have carried the diagnosis for many years [9–13]. Therefore, this study aims to find predictors of severe headache symptoms and impaired daily function in chronic IIH patients without active ophthalmological involvement.

2. Materials and Methods

2.1. Research Hypothesis

Our hypothesis was that several structural and physiological changes take place in female IIH patients. As a result, symptoms would improve with a longer duration since diagnosis. In addition, we hypothesized that lower FARB scores (indicating a more narrowed transverse-sigmoid junction) would impair venous drainage and consequently impair normal cerebrospinal fluid (CSF) drainage into the cerebral venous system. As a result, lower FARB scores would be independently associated with a higher degree of IIH symptoms and disability despite longer disease duration because ophthalmological involvement was resolved.

2.2. Statement of Ethical Approval and Consent

This study was approved by our medical institutional review board committee [number 0278-2020]. All participants consented to the anonymized use of their clinical and questionnaire data. Informed consent was obtained verbally prior to administering the questionnaire.

2.3. Study Population

We included only female IIH patients as most IIH patients are young females, and to reduce possible bias as substantial differences may exist in the underlying pathophysiology of IIH between females and males. Therefore, to be eligible for inclusion, participants had to be female, aged 18 years or older at the time of IIH diagnosis, and have cerebral venous imaging data from their initial IIH diagnosis. In addition, patients were required to have been diagnosed with IIH at least six months ago and to have been treated with CAI for at least three months prior to study enrollment. Finally, patients had to be without any signs of optic disc edema in their most recent ophthalmological evaluation. Pediatric and male patients, or patients who required surgical treatments such as a ventriculoperitoneal shunt, optic nerve fenestration, or cerebral venous stenting, were excluded from the study.

2.4. Recruitment and Sampling

Electronic medical records of patients diagnosed in our department with IIH between January 2012 and December 2018 were evaluated. Out of 210 consecutive patients, updated telephone numbers were available for 150 patients, who were called and invited to participate in the study. One-hundred-and-thirty-three patients agreed to participate in the study and complete the questionnaire. After obtaining consent, exclusion criteria were reviewed with the patients based on their electronic medical records. Consequently, 19 patients were excluded either because of the unavailability of cerebral venous imaging data from the time of IIH diagnosis or because they were undergoing a surgical procedure. The remaining 104 patients were enrolled into the study.

2.5. Data Collection

Data were collected by five different teams of researchers blinded to each other. All researchers were physicians, and special attention was given during the process of data collection to patients who required changes in their medical care. Retrospective data collection was performed by four different researchers (general medical, neurological, ophthalmological, and radiological) from the patients' index hospitalization and health medical organization (HMO) electronic medical records. Data collection was performed separately, and every researcher was blinded to the data collected by the other researchers. Additionally, to minimize possible bias, both the questionnaire and radiological review were each performed by a single researcher.

Epidemiological and general medical information including age, height, weight, and body mass index (BMI) on index hospitalization, chronic medical conditions, and medications were collected by a general physician. A neurologist ascertained the diagnosis of IIH using lumbar puncture opening pressure and CSF laboratory analysis on index admission. Ophthalmologists ascertained both the presence of either papilledema or visual field defect upon IIH diagnosis and that all participants were appropriately followed up by a neuro-ophthalmologist. Additionally, they ensured that IIH patients included in the study did not have signs of optic disc edema in their most recent ophthalmological evaluation. The questionnaire was administered within three months following the most recent ophthalmological evaluation. Imaging data were analyzed in a core laboratory by a single radiologist, who ruled out the presence of structural lesions that may contribute to increased ICP, in turn contributing to the diagnosis of IIH. The radiologist evaluated the presence of an empty sella, high jugular bulb, and slit-like ventricles, measured the optic nerve width bilaterally, and determined the dominant side of venous sinus drainage, if available. He graded transverse sinus stenosis (TSS) using the Combined Conduit Score (CCS)—an index introduced in 2003 by FARB et al. [14]. The grading of the patency is performed in each of the transverse sinuses (left and right), and the grade ranges from 0 to 4 based on the level of patency: 0—0% patency, 1—less than 25% patency, 2—25–50% patency, 3—50–75% patency, 4—75–100% patency. The score of each side is then combined to derive the CCS (0–8). A normal healthy result is 8, which signifies no or very little TSS.

2.6. Study Questionnaire

All participants enrolled in the study were interviewed between November 2020 and October 2022. The questionnaire consisted of information relating to the symptoms experienced by the participants as well as their general state of health (Supplemental Materials).

The first part of the questionnaire consisted of 35 questions concerning basic demographic characteristics, time since diagnosis, and additional medical history. The second section comprised two existing questionnaires validated for migraine patients: six questions from the Headache Impact Test (HIT-6) [15,16] for the assessment of the impact of headache on daily life and five questions from the Migraine Disability Assessment Scale (MIDAS) [17].

HIT-6 [15,16]: The Headache Impact Test-6 (HIT-6) was developed to measure a wide spectrum of factors contributing to the burden of a headache, and it has demonstrated utility for generating quantitative and pertinent information on the impact of a headache. The disability was classified using the following two impact grades based on the HIT-6 score: little-to-substantial impact (HIT-6 score: 36–59) and severe impact (HIT-6 score: >60) [15,16].

MIDAS [17]: The MIDAS is a self-reporting instrument that was administered to patients to measure headache pain intensity and headache attack frequency. Based on the total score, the severity of the migraine is classified into grades I–IV (I = little or no disability, II = mild disability, III = moderate disability, and IV = severe disability) [17].

The third part of the questionnaire focused on patients' reported outcome measures (PROMs) and included 23 questions. Satisfaction with the current medical treatment and perception of symptoms were assessed using nine questions on a scoring scale ranging from 1 ('I don't agree at all') to 5 ('Strongly agree') that included five 'Yes/No' questions. Side effects were rated using a single question, with ratings ranging from 0 ('Not at all') to 7 ('Bothers me a lot'). The last eight questions evaluated functional improvement and lifestyle changes since diagnosis (eight 'Yes/No' questions and two questions on a 1–5 scale, with '1' being 'I don't agree at all' and '5' being 'Strongly agree').

2.7. Statistical Analysis

Data analysis was performed using R software version 4.1.0 with R-Studio software version 2022.07.1. Summary statistics are presented as mean and standard deviation (SD) for continuous variables, and as numbers and percentages for binary or categorical variables. The association between every two qualitative variables was tested using the chi-square (χ^2) test. Tests between independent samples were performed using an analysis of variance (ANOVA) test after confirming that the data conformed to a normal distribution. A probability value of <0.05 was considered statistically significant, and all tests were two-sided.

The HIT and MIDAS results were analyzed as dichotomous variables. HIT: (1) Little + Mild Severity versus Moderate + Severe Severity, and MIDAS: Little + Mild Severity versus Substantial + Severe Severity (MIDAS > 55). Analysis was also performed according to the median time elapsed since the diagnosis.

Univariate analyses were used to assess differences between the above groups in demographic and clinical characteristics. Overall perception of functional difficulties in daily activities was calculated using a summary of each difficulty (ranging from 0 to 8).

3. Results

3.1. Demographics and Baseline Clinical Characteristics of Study Participants

One-hundred-and-four participants (mean age 35.5 ± 11.9 years) were diagnosed with IIH an average of 7.85 ± 7.01 years prior to participating in the study (Table 1). Ninety-two patients (88.4%) had papilledema, and 39 (37.5%) had a significant visual field defect (other than enlargement of the blind spot) upon diagnosis. One-hundred-and-four participants answered the PROMs and MIDAS questionnaire while only 102 patients answered the HIT-6 questionnaire.

Table 1. Demographic and Baseline Clinical Characteristics of Study Participants.

Characteristic	Participants (N = 104)
Age, mean (SD), y	35.6 (11.9)
BMI upon diagnosis, mean (SD), kg/m^2	34.6 (8.3)
Duration of IIH diagnosis, mean (SD), y	7.9 (7.0)
LP opening pressure at diagnosis, mean (SD), mmH$_2$O	361.0 (99.4)
Diabetes	3 (2.9)
Chronic hypertension	14 (13.6)
Polycystic ovary	19 (18.4)
Hypothyroidism	9 (8.7)
Hypertriglyceridemia	10 (9.9)
Anemia	30 (29.1)
ADHD	23 (22.3)
Depression/anxiety	16 (15.7)

Abbreviations: ADHD, attention deficit hyperactivity disorder; BMI body mass index; BP, blood pressure; IIH, idiopathic intracranial hypertension; LP, lumbar puncture.

3.2. Headache, Function, and Patient-Reported Outcome Measures (PROMs)

A high proportion of the participants reported significant difficulties in daily activities, such as watching television (31.2%) or reading (37.1%) for a long period of time, driving (25.6%), learning new information (25.5%), remembering where things were placed (38.1%), and remembering whether tasks were completed (40.2%). Furthermore, about one-third (33.9%) of the participants reported no improvement in their general physical condition, 35.8% reported difficulties in completing tasks to the best of their ability, 32% reported difficulties in keeping up with work or studies, and 39% reported a lack of happiness. Additionally, almost half of the participants (47.8%) reported feeling discouraged by the ability of the medication to treat their illness.

3.3. Medical Treatment

Twenty-nine patients (27.9%) were treated with acetazolamide or topiramate at the time of the questionnaire's administration. Of the overall study population, only 73% adhered to the instructed CAI treatment protocol. Sixty-five participants (62%) reported significant adverse effects associated with the usage of CAI. Sixty-six patients (63.4%) were dissatisfied with the effectiveness of the treatment with the medications, and over half (n = 55, 52.9%) reported taking painkillers on a regular basis to manage their chronic headaches.

3.4. Correlation between HIT-6 and MIDAS in Subgroups and Clinical Variables

Fifty-seven patients (54.8%) had a severe disability according to the MIDAS score, in contrast to 36 patients (35.3%) based on the HIT-6 score (Table S1). When comparing the little–mild (n = 58) and moderate–severe (n = 44) HIT-6 score groups, the only significant difference was a longer duration since diagnosis in the former group (9.04 ± 7.67 vs. 5.76 ± 4.89 years, $p = 0.023$) (Table S2 Supplemental Materials).

Patients with higher MIDAS disability scores (grades 3–4, n = 68), in comparison with those with lower disability scores (grades 1–2, n = 36), were younger (32.41 ± 8.93 vs. 41.47 ± 14.36, $p < 0.001$) with a significantly shorter average time since diagnosis (5.93 ± 5.27 vs. 11.73 ± 8.47 years, $p < 0.001$) (Table 2). Additionally, the FARB score was significantly lower (indicating a higher severity of narrowing in the transverse-sigmoid junction) in the high-severity MIDAS group (1.28 ± 1.82 vs. 2.87 ± 2.3, $p = 0.02$).

Table 2. Comparison between mild- versus high-severity MIDAS score groups.

MIDAS		Little-to-Mild Severity (Grade 1 + Grade 2) N = 36 (34.6%)				Moderate-to-Severe Severity (Grade 3 + Grade 4) N = 68 (65.4%)					
Variable	Subgroup	N	%	Mean	SD	N	%	Mean	SD	F/χ^2	p-Value
Age		36		41.47	14.36	68		32.41	8.93	F = 15.70	<0.001
Time since diagnosis		30		11.73	8.47	61		5.93	5.27	F = 16.08	<0.001
BMI		33		34.39	8.88	60		34.69	8.02	F = 0.03	0.87
Medical history											
Diabetes		2	5.7			1	1.5			$\chi^2 = 0.35$	0.55
Hypertension		8	22.9			6	8.8			$\chi^2 = 2.77$	0.09
Polycystic ovary		8	22.9			11	16.2			$\chi^2 = 0.31$	0.58
Hypothyroidism		2	5.7			7	10.3			$\chi^2 = 0.17$	0.68
Hypertriglyceridemia		3	8.6			7	10.6			$\chi^2 = 0$	1
Diagnosis of anxiety/depression		6	17.1			10	14.9			$\chi^2 = 0$	1
Radiology											
Empty sella		14	58.3			35	55.6			$\chi^2 = 0$	1
Slit-like vent		5	20.8			12	19			$\chi^2 = 0$	1
Flattening of sclera		11	45.8			32	50.8			$\chi^2 = 0.03$	0.86
Optic nerve sheath dilatation		18	75			46	73			$\chi^2 = 0$	1
FARB score		25		2.87	2.3	79		1.28	1.82	F = 5.57	0.02
Neuro-ophthalmology											

Table 2. Cont.

MIDAS	Subgroup	Little-to-Mild Severity (Grade 1 + Grade 2) N = 36 (34.6%)				Moderate-to-Severe Severity (Grade 3 + Grade 4) N = 68 (65.4%)				F/χ²	p-Value
Variable		N	%	Mean	SD	N	%	Mean	SD		
Papilledema at time of diagnosis		32	88.9			61	89.7			χ² = 0	1
Damage to visual fields at time of diagnosis		11	68.8			29	64.4			χ² = 0	1
Functional difficulties				3.74	2.69			5.38	3.17	F = 5.75	0.018
HIT		34				68				χ² = 57.32	<0.001
	Minimal	24	70.6			3	4.4				
	Moderate to Substantial	10	29.4			29	42.7				

Notably, a significant correlation ($\chi^2 = 57.32$, $p < 0.001$) was found between a high HIT score and a high MIDAS score, suggesting similar directionality. A logistic regression model was used to find predictors of a higher MIDAS score (Table 3).

Table 3. Multivariate model for prediction of moderate–severe MIDAS score.

Predictors	Odds Ratios	CI	p
Age	0.92	0.84–1.02	0.134
Time since diagnosis	1.05	0.84–1.23	0.931
FARB score	0.78	0.57–1.12	0.121

A negative trend was found for a higher FARB score (OR 0.78, 95% CI 0.57–1.12, $p = 0.12$). Additionally, a higher age showed a negative trend for a higher MIDAS score (OR 0.92, 95% CI 0.84–1.02, $p = 0.13$) while the time since diagnosis did not show any trend ($p = 0.93$). Fifty-seven patients were classified as severe according to the MIDAS scale, with different scores. A Pearson correlation found a tendency for an inverse correlation between the FARB severity score and the MIDAS score (-0.193, $p = 0.15$). A post hoc analysis of patients with severe MIDAS scores, comparing the 10 patients with the highest MIDAS score with the remainder of the subgroup (n = 47), found that they differed only in terms of the FARB score (1.6 ± 1.1 vs. 2.7 ± 2.4, $p = 0.041$) (Table 4).

Table 4. Sub-analysis of SEVERE MIDAS group.

Subgroup of SEVERE MIDAS	Highest Severity (n = 10)	Remainder of the SEVERE Subgroup (n = 47)	p-Value
MIDAS score $\pm$ SD	252 ± 61	84 ± 47	<0.001
Age $\pm$ SD (years)	35.6 ± 10.4	32 ± 9.2	0.266
Time from Diagnosis $\pm$ SD	6.3 ± 6.3	5.6 ± 5.4	0.735
FARB score	1.6 ± 1.1	2.7 ± 2.4	0.041

4. Discussion

In the current study, we found that headaches persist and quality of life is impaired in ophthalmologically stable female IIH patients. We focused our study on this subpopulation of females as they comprise the majority of IIH patients, and this evaluation might therefore provide further insights into the quality of the current standard of medical treatment for IIH. Our findings are supported by existing studies that similarly report persistent headaches in a significant percentage of IIH patients despite medical treatment [4,6,9,18,19].

Witry et al. [13] reported a higher ratio of patients (82%) suffering a severe impact of headaches on their daily life (HIT-6 $\geq$ 60) compared with our study (35.3%). We may attribute this high incidence to the different composition of the study populations. Our study excluded patients who were within the first 6 months after an IIH diagnosis, while they were included in the study by Witry et al. [13]. Moreover, similar results were reported by Xu et al. [6], who showed that almost half (48.8%) of the medically treated patients were still suffering from chronic headaches after an average follow-up period of 2.8 years. A 9-year observational study by Thaller et al. [9] also found a high headache burden. They found that the HIT-6 score was mildly affected by the time interval since diagnosis, and stepwise regression analysis showed that the only factors affecting long-term headache frequency were the occurrence of daily headache at diagnosis and a personal migraine history. Disease duration, change in BMI and family history of migraine were not significantly influential.

Similar to the study by Thaller et al., the multivariate logistic regression analysis in our study did not show that the time interval since IIH diagnosis had any impact on the MIDAS severity ($p = 0.93$). However, the multivariate analysis in our study showed a clear trend for younger age as a predictor of a moderate–severe MIDAS score (OR 1.09, $p = 0.13$). Possible etiologies may include age-related hormonal changes [20] and structural changes.

Our multivariate analysis found an additional interesting trend for a lower FARB score as a predictor of moderate–severe MIDAS (OR 1.3, $p = 0.12$). The 10 patients with the highest MIDAS scores were found to have the lowest FARB scores. Previous studies suggested that transverse sinus stenosis with a significant pressure gradient increases cerebral venous pressure, impairs CSF resorption in the venous system, and thereby increases intracranial (CSF) pressure, aggravating the symptoms of IIH [8,21]. To the best of our knowledge, this is the first study incorporating neuroradiology markers into the assessment of medically stable IIH patients' symptoms and QOL.

Although all the participants experienced complete resolution of their papilledema and did not suffer from a permanent and significant visual field loss with standard medical treatment, 75% experienced significant disability and very poor PROMs. Moreover, 15.7% of the study participants were formally diagnosed with depression or anxiety. Multiple studies have also reported high rates of anxiety and depression in chronic IIH patients, as well as significant disability and poor quality of life (QoL) [6,13,22–26]. Other works found cognitive impairment in multiple domains (e.g., impaired networks (executive function) and sustained attention) in female adult IIH patients compared with controls [16]. Biousse and Newman showed the multidisciplinary manifestations of IIH, which results in visual loss, chronic headaches, chronic tinnitus, depression, and even cognitive impairment, with decreased quality of life and chronic disability being associated with multiple hospital admissions. They concluded that there is a pressing need for a better understanding and improved management of IIH to limit the inevitable burden on healthcare systems around the world. The authors suggested a multidisciplinary, holistic approach to the treatment of IIH, addressing all aspects of the expanding spectrum of IIH and targeting not only direct treatment of intracranial hypertension and papilledema but also aggressive management of headache, CSF leak repair, symptomatic relief, improvement of patient quality of life, and sustained weight loss.

In this cohort, we noticed an improvement in disease symptoms over time, possibly due to age-related changes. Part of the improvement seen in the older IIH patients may have been influenced by the reduction in migraine severity among menopausal women. Our study did not differentiate between headache types, and we therefore could not fully investigate that possibility. Nevertheless, even 10 years after diagnosis, eight participants (7.6% of the entire cohort) had moderate-to-severe MIDAS scores. Our study adds to the current literature supporting the idea that IIH remains chronic in a significant number of patients and that the currently available medications mainly target the ophthalmologic aspect of the disease. From the patients' perspective, despite the improvement of ophthalmologic symptoms, almost half (47.8%) of our study participants felt discouraged by the ability of medications to treat their illness.

Most of our study cohort was treated with acetazolamide (87%), and the remaining participants were treated with topiramate. In total, 16 of 104 (15.38%) patients reported severe adverse effects attributed to the medications they were given. Severe adverse effects, mainly related to acetazolamide, are well described in the literature [4,6,13,19,27]. Xu et al. [6] reported that during a 1-year follow-up period, 34.2% of the patients stopped the usage of acetazolamide, and 36.4% stopped topiramate due to adverse events. The rate of adherence to acetazolamide during 6 months of the NORDIC trial [7] was 89%, which is better than that reported by Xu et al. [6]. but still reflects difficulties in coping with long-term drug treatment.

In our study, 55/104 (52.9%) patients reported taking painkillers on a routine basis. The routine use of painkillers leading to a degree of overuse has been described in multiple studies. Similar results were presented in a review study by Mollan et al. [23] showing the regular use of analgesic medications in up to half of IIH patients, depending on the study.

As in prior studies, no correlation was found in our study between the severity of pain or disability and the BMI, opening pressure on lumbar puncture, medical background, or papilledema at diagnosis [18,28]. We did not identify any radiological findings that could be used as potential predictors of disability or headache severity, apart from the FARB score. Additionally, we did not find any other studies in the literature that evaluated similar radiological findings as potential predictors for comparison purposes.

Our study demonstrated significant disability (MIDAS), headache (HIT-6), and PROMs in chronic IIH patients treated with medications, even years post-diagnosis. Different studies that investigated the HIT-6 and MIDAS scores, as well as other scores related to QoL, also showed a significant disease burden. Currently, there are no disease-specific validated tools to evaluate QoL and other disease-related symptoms in IIH patients [22]. Until such a tool is available or a large multicenter study is performed, it will be difficult to assess the extent of the disease burden in IIH and hence the efficacy of the current standard treatment.

The currently available medications for the treatment of IIH have not been proven to be efficient for all disease aspects in longitudinal studies. Many studies indicated a high rate of significant adverse effects, which may affect the treatment compliance and may worsen the QoL. We found lower HIT-6 and MIDAS scores in patients diagnosed a relatively long time prior to study participation.

Our study has several limitations. The aim of our study was to evaluate the long-term headache and functional outcomes in ophthalmologically resolved women with IIH. Unfortunately, we did not find well-validated scales for this evaluation in IIH patients. As a result, we chose to include both the MIDAS and HIT-6 in our questionnaire, which are scales validated for migraine patients and not for IIH patients. Notably, our sample size was small, with only 104 patients being included. Another important limitation is the retrospective nature of part of the data collection. Moreover, the questionnaire was administered only once to each patient. Finally, our cross-sectional study did not include questions regarding the phenotype of headaches (characteristics of migraine, tension headache, or both). This is important because Thaller et al. found that the two main factors influencing high headache frequency and worse prognosis were a personal migraine history and daily headache at baseline [9]. Prospective studies with larger samples are required to understand treatment outcomes in IIH patients.

5. Conclusions

Similar to previous studies, our study using a detailed questionnaire found that IIH symptoms persist, and quality of life is impaired, even years after ophthalmological stability has been achieved in IIH female patients. We found in our multivariate model that a higher FARB score and older age showed a negative trend for higher severity according to the MIDAS scale score. Finally, the 10 patients with the highest MIDAS severity scores differed from the remainder of the patients with severe MIDAS scores only by having lower FARB scores. Thus, we assume that severe IIH symptomology may be impacted by a narrowing of the transverse sigmoid sinus junction. We regard our findings as hypothesis-generating only, and further large scale, consecutive, prospective imaging-based studies are therefore needed to understand the long-standing symptoms of female IIH patients.

Supplementary Materials: The following supporting information can be downloaded at: https://www.mdpi.com/article/10.3390/jcm13133971/s1, Table S1: Degree of Disability in the Study Population as Assessed Using the Headache Impact Test (HIT-6) and the Migraine Disability Assessment (MIDAS) Scores; Table S2: Comparison Between Participants by HIT-6 scores (Little to Mild versus Moderate to Severe).

Author Contributions: A.H. (Asaf Honig): writing—original and final draft, validation, formal analysis, and visualization. A.H. (Anat Horev) and A.H. (Asaf Honig): conceptualization, methodology, writing—review and editing, and supervision. M.K. and R.B.: statistical analysis. A.H. (Anat Horev), S.A.-B., E.T., T.R., M.K., G.I., R.B., Y.Z., G.B.-A., and I.S.: data curation. T.E.: writing—review and editing. All authors contributed to the article and approved the submitted version. All authors have read and agreed to the published version of the manuscript.

Funding: The authors declare that no funds, grants, or other support were received during the preparation of this manuscript.

Institutional Review Board Statement: This study was approved by our medical institutional review board committee [number 0278-2020] on 15 December 2016 and valid until 14 December 2015. All participants consented to the anonymized use of their clinical data, as well as to the additional questionnaire data being collected and analyzed. Informed consent was obtained verbally prior to answering the questionnaire. Patients were assured confidentiality, and the questionnaire was conducted according to the American Medical Association's ethical standards for conducting a questionnaire survey.

Informed Consent Statement: Informed consent was obtained from all subjects involved in the study.

Data Availability Statement: The original contributions presented in the study are included in the article; further inquiries can be directed to the corresponding author.

Conflicts of Interest: The authors declare that the research was conducted in the absence of any commercial or financial relationships that could be construed as potential conflicts of interest.

References

1. Friedman, D.I.; Liu, G.T.; Digre, K.B. Revised diagnostic criteria for the pseudotumor cerebri syndrome in adults and children. *Neurology* **2013**, *81*, 1159–1165. [CrossRef] [PubMed]
2. Wall, M. Idiopathic intracranial hypertension. *Neurol. Clin.* **1991**, *9*, 73–95. [CrossRef]
3. Mollan, S.P.; Mytton, J.; Tsermoulas, G.; Sinclair, A.J. Idiopathic Intracranial Hypertension: Evaluation of Admissions and Emergency Readmissions through the Hospital Episode Statistic Dataset between 2002–2020. *Life* **2021**, *11*, 417. [CrossRef] [PubMed]
4. Ball, A.K.; Howman, A.; Wheatley, K.; Burdon, M.A.; Matthews, T.; Jacks, A.S.; Lawden, M.; Sivaguru, A.; Furmston, A.; Howell, S.; et al. A randomised controlled trial of treatment for idiopathic intracranial hypertension. *J. Neurol.* **2011**, *258*, 874–881. [CrossRef] [PubMed]
5. Raoof, N.; Hoffmann, J. Diagnosis and treatment of idiopathic intracranial hypertension. *Cephalalgia* **2021**, *41*, 472–478. [CrossRef] [PubMed]
6. Xu, W.; Prime, Z.; Papchenko, T.; Danesh-Meyer, H.V. Long term outcomes of idiopathic intracranial hypertension: Observational study and literature review. *Clin. Neurol. Neurosurg.* **2021**, *205*, 106463. [CrossRef] [PubMed]
7. Wall, M.; McDermott, M.P.; Kieburtz, K.D.; Corbett, J.J.; Feldon, S.E.; Friedman, D.I.; Katz, D.M.; Keltner, J.L.; Schron, E.B.; Kupersmith, M.J. Effect of acetazolamide on visual function in patients with idiopathic intracranial hypertension and mild visual loss: The idiopathic intracranial hypertension treatment trial. *JAMA* **2014**, *311*, 1641–1651. [CrossRef] [PubMed]
8. Ahmed, R.M.; Wilkinson, M.; Parker, G.D.; Thurtell, M.J.; Macdonald, J.; McCluskey, P.J.; Allan, R.; Dunne, V.; Hanlon, M.; Owler, B.K.; et al. Transverse sinus stenting for idiopathic intracranial hypertension: A review of 52 patients and of model predictions. *AJNR Am. J. Neuroradiol.* **2011**, *32*, 1408–1414. [CrossRef] [PubMed]
9. Thaller, M.; Homer, V.; Hyder, Y.; Yiangou, A.; Liczkowski, A.; Fong, A.W.; Virdee, J.; Piccus, R.; Roque, M.; Mollan, S.P.; et al. The idiopathic intracranial hypertension prospective cohort study: Evaluation of prognostic factors and outcomes. *J. Neurol.* **2023**, *270*, 851–863. [CrossRef]
10. Micieli, J.A.; Gorham, J.P.; Bruce, B.B.; Newman, N.J.; Biousse, V.; Peragallo, J.H. Clinical and demographic differences between idiopathic intracranial hypertension patients with mild and severe papilledema. *Taiwan. J. Ophthalmol.* **2021**, *11*, 53–56. [CrossRef]
11. Hatem, C.F.; Yri, H.M.; Sørensen, A.L.; Wegener, M.; Jensen, R.H.; Hamann, S. Long-term visual outcome in a Danish population of patients with idiopathic intracranial hypertension. *Acta Ophthalmol.* **2018**, *96*, 719–723. [CrossRef] [PubMed]
12. Behbehani, R.; Ali, A.; Al-Moosa, A. Course and Predictors of Visual Outcome of Idiopathic Intracranial Hypertension. *Neuroophthalmology* **2022**, *46*, 80–84. [CrossRef] [PubMed]
13. Witry, M.; Kindler, C.; Weller, J.; Linder, A.; Wüllner, U. The patients perspective on the burden of idiopathic intracranial hypertension. *J. Headache Pain* **2021**, *22*, 67. [CrossRef] [PubMed]
14. Farb, R.I.; Vanek, I.; Scott, J.N.; Mikulis, D.J.; Willinsky, R.A.; Tomlinson, G.; terBrugge, K.G. Idiopathic intracranial hypertension: The prevalence and morphology of sinovenous stenosis. *Neurology* **2003**, *60*, 1418–1424. [CrossRef] [PubMed]
15. Bayliss, M.S.; Dewey, J.E.; Dunlap, I.; Batenhorst, A.S.; Cady, R.; Diamond, M.L.; Sheftell, F. A study of the feasibility of Internet administration of a computerized health survey: The headache impact test (HIT). *Qual. Life Res.* **2003**, *12*, 953–961. [CrossRef] [PubMed]
16. Kosinski, M.; Bayliss, M.S.; Bjorner, J.B.; Ware, J.E., Jr.; Garber, W.H.; Batenhorst, A.; Cady, R.; Dahlöf, C.G.; Dowson, A.; Tepper, S. A six-item short-form survey for measuring headache impact: The HIT-6. *Qual. Life Res.* **2003**, *12*, 963–974. [CrossRef] [PubMed]
17. Stewart, W.F.; Lipton, R.B.; Dowson, A.J.; Sawyer, J. Development and testing of the Migraine Disability Assessment (MIDAS) Questionnaire to assess headache-related disability. *Neurology* **2001**, *56*, S20–S28. [CrossRef] [PubMed]

18. Friedman, D.I.; Quiros, P.A.; Subramanian, P.S.; Mejico, L.J.; Gao, S.; McDermott, M.; Wall, M. Headache in Idiopathic Intracranial Hypertension: Findings From the Idiopathic Intracranial Hypertension Treatment Trial. *Headache* **2017**, *57*, 1195–1205. [CrossRef] [PubMed]
19. Yri, H.M.; Rönnbäck, C.; Wegener, M.; Hamann, S.; Jensen, R.H. The course of headache in idiopathic intracranial hypertension: A 12-month prospective follow-up study. *Eur. J. Neurol.* **2014**, *21*, 1458–1464. [CrossRef]
20. Hoyos-Martinez, A.; Horne, V.E.; Wood, A.C.; Shah, V. Prevalence of Adrenal Insufficiency and Glucocorticoid Use in Pediatric Pseudotumor Cerebri Syndrome. *J. Neuroophthalmol.* **2021**, *41*, e451–e457. [CrossRef]
21. Horev, A.; Ben-Arie, G.; Walter, E.; Tsumi, E.; Regev, T.; Aloni, E.; Biederko, R.; Zlotnik, Y.; Lebowitz, Z.; Shelef, I.; et al. Emergent cerebral venous stenting: A valid treatment option for fulminant idiopathic intracranial hypertension. *J. Neurol. Sci.* **2023**, *452*, 120761. [CrossRef] [PubMed]
22. Mollan, S.P.; Sinclair, A.J. Outcomes measures in idiopathic intracranial hypertension. *Expert. Rev. Neurother.* **2021**, *21*, 687–700. [CrossRef] [PubMed]
23. Mollan, S.P.; Grech, O.; Sinclair, A.J. Headache attributed to idiopathic intracranial hypertension and persistent post-idiopathic intracranial hypertension headache: A narrative review. *Headache* **2021**, *61*, 808–816. [CrossRef] [PubMed]
24. Raggi, A.; Marzoli, S.B.; Chiapparini, L.; Ciasca, P.; Erbetta, A.; Faragò, G.; Grazzi, L.; Leonardi, M.; D'Amico, D. Headache frequency and symptoms of depression as predictors of disability in patients with idiopathic intracranial hypertension. *Neurol. Sci.* **2018**, *39* (Suppl. 1), 139–140. [CrossRef] [PubMed]
25. de Oliveira, M.F.; Yamashita, R.H.G.; Boa Sorte, A.A., Jr.; Rotta, J.M.; Norremose, K.A.; Teixeira, M.J.; Pinto, F.C.G. Psychiatric symptoms are frequent in idiopathic intracranial hypertension patients. *Neurosurg. Rev.* **2021**, *44*, 1183–1189. [CrossRef] [PubMed]
26. Kleinschmidt, J.J.; Digre, K.B.; Hanover, R. Idiopathic intracranial hypertension: Relationship to depression, anxiety, and quality of life. *Neurology* **2000**, *54*, 319–324. [CrossRef] [PubMed]
27. Mollan, S.P.; Markey, K.A.; Benzimra, J.D.; Jacks, A.; Matthews, T.D.; Burdon, M.A.; Sinclair, A.J. A practical approach to, diagnosis, assessment and management of idiopathic intracranial hypertension. *Pract. Neurol.* **2014**, *14*, 380–390. [CrossRef]
28. Schaller, B. Physiology of cerebral venous blood flow: From experimental data in animals to normal function in humans. *Brain Res. Rev.* **2004**, *46*, 243–260. [CrossRef]

Disclaimer/Publisher's Note: The statements, opinions and data contained in all publications are solely those of the individual author(s) and contributor(s) and not of MDPI and/or the editor(s). MDPI and/or the editor(s) disclaim responsibility for any injury to people or property resulting from any ideas, methods, instructions or products referred to in the content.

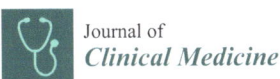

Article

Efficacy of Desvenlafaxine in Reducing Migraine Frequency and Severity: A Retrospective Study

Marina Stoupa Hadidi [1], Murad Rasheed [2], Yanal M. Bisharat [3], Heba H. Al Helou [3], Hussam A. El Aina [4], Hala M. Batayneh [4], Alaa A. A. Aljabali [5] and Omar Gammoh [6,*]

[1] Jordan Hospital, Adib Wehbeh St., Amman 11152, Jordan; marinahadidi@gmail.com
[2] The Specialty Hospital, Hunayn Bin Ishak St, Amman 11193, Jordan; murad_rasheed@yahoo.com
[3] Medical Affairs Department, MS Pharma Regional Office, Zahran Plaza Bldg., 7th Circle Amman, Amman 11844, Jordan; yanal.bisharat@mspharma.com (Y.M.B.); heba.alhelou@mspharma.com (H.H.A.H.)
[4] Marketing Department, MS Pharma Regional Office, Zahran Plaza Bldg., 7th Circle Amman, Amman 11844, Jordan; hussam.alaina@mspharma.com (H.A.E.A.); hala.batayneh@mspharma.com (H.M.B.)
[5] Department of Pharmaceutics and Pharmaceutical Technology, Yarmouk University, Irbid 21163, Jordan; alaaj@yu.edu.jo
[6] Department of Clinical Pharmacy and Pharmacy Practice, Faculty of Pharmacy, Yarmouk University, Irbid 21163, Jordan
* Correspondence: omar.gammoh@yu.edu.jo

Abstract: Background: Migraine is characterized by sudden acute episodes of pain, with a global prevalence of 18% among all age groups. It is the second leading cause of years lived with disability worldwide. Prophylactic treatment is important in managing migraine; however, its efficacy and safety are debated. This study aimed to evaluate the efficacy of desvenlafaxine in female patients with migraine. **Methods:** We conducted a retrospective observational case study involving 10 women diagnosed with migraine who were treated with desvenlafaxine. We measured the number of migraine days per month, average headache duration in minutes, headache severity using a visual analog scale, use of acute medications, and frequency of acute medication use per week. **Results:** Desvenlafaxine significantly reduced the number of migraine days from 14.70 ± 3.68 at baseline to 2.50 ± 2.50 at follow-up ($p < 0.05$). The average headache duration dropped from 131.25 ± 32.81 min to 52.50 ± 44.64 min. Headache severity scores improved from 6.80 ± 1.49 at baseline to 0.80 ± 0.92 at follow up, the frequency of acute medication use per week reduced from 3.30 ± 1.49 at baseline to 0.80 ± 0.92, and the frequency of acute medication use decreased from 3.30 ± 1.49 times per week to 0.80 ± 0.92. **Conclusions:** Desvenlafaxine shows potential as an effective prophylactic therapy for migraine. Larger-scale studies are necessary to further explore its benefits.

Keywords: desvenlafaxine; migraine; prophylaxis; pain; women; episodes; headache; frequency; severity; disability

1. Introduction

Migraine is a worldwide disabling neurological disorder featuring severe headaches that affects more than 10% of the general population [1]. Migraine presents in women more than in men; according to current estimations, 12% of women versus 6% of men are diagnosed with migraine [2], leading to professional and social disabilities [3]. Migraine attacks may last for hours or even days. They come with awful pain, nausea, and sensitivity to light and sound. This means losing workdays and time. Individuals suffering become less productive and experience impaired social and professional life.

The research on migraine in women is deeply rooted. Migraine was shown to almost always prevail in women at higher rates than men; for example, one study underscored that women were diagnosed with migraine twice as often as men [1,4]. Moreover, according to the estimations, migraine attacks were higher in females; several studies confirmed that women could suffer from more than one attack per month [1,5]. This fact also explains the higher number of physicians visit due to migraine; one study demonstrated that women account for almost 80% of migraine physicians visits [6].

According to the literature and clinical experience, people with migraine do not only suffer from the experience of migraines; the worst consequence is the continuous worry about the next migraine episode, including its intensity, timing, and duration. This presents these patients with a higher risk of psychological burden, which significantly affects their behavior and quality of life. For instance, some patients could have increased anxiety, social avoidance, and disruption of their social relationships and jobs [7,8]. According to the estimations of the Global Burden of Disease in 2016, migraine was labeled as the second leading cause of years lived with disability [9,10]. Therefore, the socioeconomic burden of migraine is an important nexus that warrants investigation. In Germany, for example, a recent analysis comprising >15 million migraine patients revealed that the annual socioeconomic losses for migraine are estimated to be EUR 100.4 billion [8]

According to the literature, migraine headaches and depression are highly associated [11,12]. This can be attributed to genetic factors, environmental factors, and stress, which activate catecholamines such as serotonin and norepinephrine. In general, the role of serotonin is evident in migraine headache pathophysiology; migraine is associated with low serotonin levels, especially between attacks [13].

Migraine pathophysiology represents a complex interplay between numerous neurotransmitters, proteins, enzymes, and genes. The role of serotonin (5-hydroxytryptamine (5-HT)) in migraine has been studied for decades. The serotonergic system projects nearly to all the different regions of the brain, including the sensory cortex, the thalamus, and the dorsal horns of the spinal cord, and is involved in many functions related to pain modulation, cortical sensory processing, and others based on its interaction with its different receptors [14–18]. Early evidence suggests the involvement of circulating serotonin in migraine. One very early investigation demonstrated that serotonin levels were significantly higher in people with migraine compared to their healthy peers during migraine attacks. These high levels, however, were normalized between attacks; this could be due to the intense enzymatic degradation by monoamine oxidases [19,20]. Even earlier evidence pointed towards an increased urinary excretion of a major metabolite of serotonin, 5-hydroxy indole acetic acid, during migraine attacks [13]. These clinical findings could establish a trend that highlights that people with migraine have low serotonin levels that spike during the attacks. In addition, in vivo studies have demonstrated a significant role of norepinephrine in the inhibition of neuropathic pain [21]. Central pain modulation is mediated by the midbrain periaqueductal grey matter. This pain modulation mechanism is stimulated by the enkephalin-releasing neurons that, in turn, activate the rostral ventromedial medulla, which in turn releases serotonin and norepinephrine, gamma-aminobutyric acid, and other mediators [22,23]. Mediations that can interfere with the release of these medications can have analgesic effects [22,24].

The endogenous descending pain inhibitory system, stemming from the rostral ventral medulla to the spinal cord, is mainly activated by norepinephrine [25,26]. Therefore, maintaining high post-synaptic levels of norepinephrine, and, to a lesser extent, serotonin, results in a sustained activation of the descending pain inhibitory pathway [27,28]. This can be achieved by using medications that inhibit the transporters of norepinephrine and serotonin such as tricyclic antidepressants and serotonin-norepinephrine reuptake inhibitors.

This supports the plethora of previous studies highlighting the roles of amitriptyline and venlafaxine in migraine prophylaxis, underscoring the implication of serotonin and norepinephrine in migraine [29,30]. Published studies indicate that dopamine and glutamate may contribute to migraine pathophysiology. This can also explain why people report very different symptoms. Very different triggers activate them. This is due to the complex interplay of these neurotransmitters [31,32].

The availability of a wide range of prophylactic therapy for patients with migraine is crucial because it improves the daily functioning and the quality of life of patients and reduces the consumption of acute analgesics and other related medications [33]. Despite the approval of several prophylactic therapies for migraine headaches, such as beta-blockers and antiepileptic medications, the evaluation of antidepressants such as serotonin-norepinephrine reuptake inhibitors (SNRIs) widens the therapeutic options for clinicians as SNRIs are preferred over TCAs due to their higher safety profile, mainly related to the cardiovascular and anticholinergic side effects [34].

The current prophylactic treatments for migraine include beta-blockers, antiepileptics, antidepressants, and biological treatments [35,36]. All these medications have their own efficacy profiles and side effects. These reported results show the need for diverse treatment options. Desvenlafaxine, a well-known potent and effective SNRI, is used in major depression disorder and demonstrated efficacy in improving neuropathic pain symptoms. Desvenlafaxine, the primary active metabolite of venlafaxine, is administered as desvenlafaxine succinate and is usually well-tolerated at a dose range of 50–100 mg/day [37]. Higher doses, reaching up to 400 mg/day, were still tolerated and effective in diabetic neuropathy [38,39]. According to the literature, no previous reports demonstrated the potential benefit of desvenlafaxine in improving migraine outcomes in female patients with migraine. One very recent study reported desvenlafaxine efficacy in migraine prophylaxis [40]. Therefore, the present case series aims to provide a preliminary evaluation of desvenlafaxine as a potential prophylactic therapy for females with migraine. Desvenlafaxine helps in treating depression and nerve pain. It has fewer side effects compared to tricyclic antidepressants. As such, it may be a good option for preventing migraines. This drug has two effects, acting on both the serotonin and norepinephrine systems. These imbalances mirror those seen in patients with migraine [41].

2. Materials and Methods

2.1. The Study Design and Settings

This is an observational study that used medical charts of patients retrospectively. It allowed us to evaluate real clinical data over a longer period. The patients were selected from two private neurology clinics in Amman, the capital of Jordan. Both clinics serve large cities. Most migraine patients are resident in those cities. Clinics were selected based on this criterion. They were chosen because they specialized in treating headache disorders. They also used the same diagnostic criterion for migraine. The data collection took place in March and April 2024. We chose this timeframe to allow for adequate follow-up periods, which are needed to assess treatment outcomes. The study was approved by Yarmouk University IRB (094/2024). The clinicians obtained consent from the patients to use their data for scientific purposes, and all data were kept anonymous.

2.2. Inclusion Criteria

Only females, using desvenlafaxine (Davlex®, United pharmaceuticals, Amman, Jordan) for at least one month, aged above 18 years, diagnosed with migraine after detailed medical history and neurological examination, and with normal brain MRI were included in the study. The exclusion criteria included: pregnancy, lactation, and other conditions linked to chronic pain. It also included treatment with other antidepressants or migraine medications. The study duration was six months. Participants recorded migraine frequency, intensity, and duration in headache diaries. Desvenlafaxine's efficacy was measured by MIDAS before starting therapy. It was measured again at the end of the study.

2.3. Study Instrument

A well-structured study instrument was created to collect information about the patients. The demographics comprised age, smoking status, and employment status. The clinical information included family history of migraine, the presence or absence of any comorbidities with migraine, the duration of migraine diagnosis, migraine headache type (episodic, or chronic), brain MRI, and the dose and duration of Davlex®.

2.4. Outcome Measurement

Migraine severity was the primary outcome measure of the study. This was evaluated using five structured questions, as in previous literature [34]: Number of migraine days per month, the average headache duration in minutes, Headache severity visual analog scale (0–10), the use of acute medication, and the frequency of acute medication use per week. These measures were taken at the baseline and at the follow-up visits by the therapist.

2.5. Data Analysis

Descriptive data of the demographic and clinical data were depicted for each of the 10 cases. In addition, the paired t-test was used to examine the difference in the mean scores of the outcome variable (migraine) between the baseline and the follow-up visit. Confidence intervals were set at 95% and significance at $p < 0.05$. Data were presented as mean $\pm$ Standard deviation (SD). Data were analyzed using SPSS software version 21.

3. Results

3.1. Study Sample Characteristics

Data were analyzed from 10 female patients diagnosed with migraine. The patients' ages ranged between 22 and 50 years old. Nine out of ten patients were non-smokers, eight were unemployed, six did not have a family history of migraine, and all the patients reported normal brain MRI. The collected data on patient histories included migraine frequency and severity and response to treatment. It also considered potential triggers. These included anxiety and depression. This provided a more comprehensive understanding of the patient's migraine profile. Please refer to Table 1 for detailed patient information.

Table 1. The description of the patient's demographics and clinical information.

	Age (Years)	Smoking Status	Employment Status	Chronic Conditions	Family History of Migraine	Migraine Diagnosis Since	Migraine Type	Normal Brain MRI
Case 1	49	Non-smoker	Unemployed	Anemia	No	5 years	Chronic	Yes
Case 2	35	Non-smoker	Unemployed		Yes	15 years	Episodic	Yes
Case 3	29	Non-smoker	Unemployed	Anxiety	No	3 years	Episodic	Yes
Case 4	46	Non-smoker	Unemployed		No	12 years	Episodic	Yes
Case 5	50	Non-smoker	Unemployed	Type II diabetes, fibromyalgia	No	3 years	Chronic	Yes
Case 6	50	Non-smoker	Unemployed	Hypertension	No	2 years	Chronic	Yes
Case 7	42	Non-smoker	Employed		Yes	10 years	Chronic	Yes
Case 8	49	Non-smoker	Employed	Shoulder Arthritis	Yes	4 years	Chronic	Yes
Case 9	45	Smoker	Unemployed		No	8 years	Chronic	Yes
Case 10	22	Non-smoker	Unemployed		Yes	6 months	Chronic	Yes

3.2. Migraine Assessment

Table 2 provides a detailed description of the number of migraine days per month, headache duration in minutes, headache severity visual analog scale (0–10), the required acute medication, the frequency of acute medication use per week, and the side effects of each of the cases. Parameters such as these give the trend of migraine attacks and treatment efficacy. It also shows variations in how individuals respond to the laid-down strategies. These strategies are for managing migraines. This information is vital as it is used to tailor treatment plans for better patient outcomes.

Table 2. Migraine assessment at baseline and follow-up visit per each case.

Cases on DSV (Desvenlafaxine)	Time Points	Number of Migraine Days per Month	Headache Duration in Minutesh	Headache severity Visual Analogue Scale (0–10)	Required Acute Medication	Frequency of Acute Medication Use/Week	Side Effects Reported
Case 1: DSV 50 mg for 2 months	Baseline	16	120	7	Yes	5	
	Follow-up	5	90	4	Yes	2	
Case 2: DSV 100 mg for 1 month	Baseline	12	120	6	Yes	2	
	Follow-up	0	0	0	No	0	
Case 3: DSV: maintenance 100 mg for 5 months	Baseline	12	180	6	Yes	5	
	Follow-up	4	90	6	Yes	1	
Case 4: DSV: maintenance 100 mg for 1 month	Baseline	10	120	7	Yes	4	
	Follow-up	5	90	4	Yes	2	
Case 5: DSV: maintenance 100 mg for 3 months	Baseline	15	120	7	Yes	2	
	Follow-up	6	90	5	Yes	1	
Case 6: DSV: maintenance 100 mg for 10 months	Baseline	20	180	7	Yes	4	
	Follow-up	0	0	0	None	0	
Case 7: DSV maintenance 100 mg for 3 months, returned to 50 mg	Baseline	17	120	6	Yes	2	Constipation on 100 mg
	Follow-up	1	60	4	None	0	
Case 8: DSV maintenance 100 mg for 12 months, returned to 50 mg	Baseline	15	90	7	Yes	1	
	Follow-up	0	0	0	None	0	
Case 9: DSV maintenance 100 mg for 16 months	Baseline	20	Almost all day long	8	Yes	5	
	Follow-up	4	120	4	Yes	2	
Case 10: DSV maintenance 50 mg for 6 months	Baseline	10	Almost all day long	7	Yes	3	
	Follow-up	0	0	0	0	0	

Table 3 demonstrates the paired t-test analysis to compare the migraine severity at baseline and the follow-up visit after using desvenlafaxine. For example, the number of migraine days per month at baseline (14.70 ± 3.68) was significantly reduced at the follow-up (2.50 ± 2.50), ((t = 8.54, 9), $p < 0.001$). Also, headache duration in minutes at baseline (131.25 ± 32.81) was significantly reduced at the follow-up (52.50 ± 44.64) ((t = 4.20, 7), $p = 0.004$). Headache severity visual analog scale at baseline (6.80 ± 0.63) was reduced significantly at the follow-up (2.70 ± 2.40) ((t = 5.16, 9), $p = 0.001$)), and the frequency of acute medication use per week at baseline (3.30 ± 1.49) was significantly reduced at the follow-up (0.80 ± 0.92), ((t = 7.32, 9), $p < 0.001$). This is a significant improvement in the syndrome of migraines. It also cuts the need for acute medication after using desvenlafaxine. The statistical analysis is significant. It shows that desvenlafaxine reduces migraines' frequency, duration, and severity.

In summary, the results demonstrate that desvenlafaxine was able to significantly reduce all the outcome variables investigated, namely, the number of migraine days per month, the average headache duration in minutes, the headache severity on the visual analog scale, and the frequency of acute medication use per week.

Table 3. Paired-*t*-test analysis for the migraine outcome measurements.

	Baseline Mean ± SD	Follow-Up Mean ± SD	t, df	*p*-Value
Number of migraine days per month	14.70 ± 3.68	2.50 ± 2.50	8.54, 9	<0.001 *
Headache duration in minutes	131.25 ± 32.81	52.50 ± 44.64	4.20, 7	0.004 *
Headache severity visual analogue scale (0–10)	6.80 ± 0.63	2.70 ± 2.40	5.16, 9	0.001 *
Frequency of acute medication use/week	3.30 ± 1.49	0.80 ± 0.92	7.32, 9	<0.001 *

SD: standard deviation, t: *t*-test score, df: degrees of freedom, * $p < 0.05$.

4. Discussion

Migraine is a widespread disorder featuring moderate to severe unilateral pain episodes that can last from 4 h to 3 consecutive days. This is often accompanied by other symptoms such as nausea, vomiting, pallor, fatigue, lack of concentration, photophobia, diarrhea, and others [42]. The pathophysiological basis of migraine pain is neurogenic inflammation and vasodilation in the meninges, which leads to the sensitization of the nociceptive afferents [43]. While acute analgesics are recommended for all people with migraine, use of prophylaxis is an essential strategy for several patients. This study tried to explore the potential of using desvenlafaxine in migraine prophylaxis to provide clinicians with another therapeutic option that can extend the list of available prophylactic medications. Our results from this small-scale study of 10 cases demonstrated promising results. Desvenlafaxine was able to diminish the number of migraine days per month, the average headache duration in minutes, the headache severity on the visual analog scale, and the frequency of acute medication use per week.

According to an evidence-based comprehensive review [36], the prophylactic therapies are grouped according to their postulated efficacy and side effects as follows: Group 1: moderate to highly effective with infrequent side effects, including amitriptyline and valproate. Group 2: Lower efficacy than group 1, and mild to moderate side effects, including aspirin, gabapentin, and atenolol. Group 3: effective prophylactic medications that lack substantial evidence, such as bupropion and diltiazem. Group 4: Medium to high efficacy medications, good strength of evidence, but with side effect concerns, such as flunarizine. Group 5: medications with no efficacy in migraine prophylaxis, such as carbamazepine.

The ultimate goal of prophylactic therapy is to both reduce the number and the severity of the episode and therefore improve the quality of life of the patients and enhance their daily functioning. Recently, besides the clinical efficacy, patient satisfaction and willingness to start prophylactic therapy have also been taken into consideration [1,42,44].

Researchers believe that desvenlafaxine provides extensive relief for migraine sufferers. This is because it cuts migraine days. It also reduces the length and severity of headaches and it lowers the use of acute medication. Improvements in all these measures show desvenlafaxine's potential to improve patients' lives. It also reduces the burden of migraines.

Our finding is consistent with the only available previous study [40], where desvenlafaxine demonstrated efficacy in migraine prophylaxis. Although the entire mechanism is not fully understood, based on existing evidence, this effect has been attributed to the 5-HT and NE reuptake mechanism of desvenlafaxine, which is the same mechanism found in venlafaxine and amitriptyline, the famous tricyclic antidepressant [45–47]. Clinical experience supports this explanation. Amitriptyline has been used for chronic pain for decades, and it has also been employed in migraine prophylaxis [48,49]. Desvenlafaxine acts on serotonin and norepinephrine. This may also help it work to prevent migraines. Serotonin helps to modulate pain and regulate blood vessel tension, while norepinephrine helps with pain perception and autonomic nervous system function. Desvenlafaxine may stabilize migraine-related neural pathways by modulating key neurotransmitter systems.

On the other hand, due to the side effects profile of amitriptyline, which includes cardiovascular side effects, sedation, postural hypotension, dry mouth, and histaminergic effects [50,51], its use has declined and it has been replaced by venlafaxine, a newer SNRI medication that shares the same mechanism but comes with higher tolerability [52].

Desvenlafaxine, the principal metabolite of venlafaxine, is understudied in migraine prophylaxis. Venlafaxine, however, has been extensively studied in migraine prophylaxis. For example, venlafaxine was shown to decrease the mean number of headaches per month starting from the first month of treatment and reaching maximum effects in 6–7 months of use. Venlafaxine also improved the reported global efficacy in about 88% of patients with migraine [53,54]. The efficacy of venlafaxine is dose-related as higher doses ensure higher inhibition of neuronal NE reuptake [54]. However, according to some studies, about 18% of patients discontinued venlafaxine due to side effects that could be dose-related [53]. In our study, desvenlafaxine worked as well as venlafaxine did in past studies. However, its simpler metabolism and once-a-day dosing may make desvenlafaxine more effective. It may lead to better patient compliance and less potential for drug-drug interactions. More studies are needed to compare venlafaxine and desvenlafaxine for preventing migraines. These studies will help us understand their effectiveness and tolerability. Desvenlafaxine's effects on migraine would have been outside of serotonin and norepinephrine's influence. For example, it could ease the cortical spreading of depression. This is a key part of migraine with aura. Additionally, it could block neurogenic inflammation and the influence of calcitonin gene-related peptides. These have been linked to migraine pain. Research into these supposed mechanisms may better explain their role.

Migraine prophylaxis research is beset by challenges in different aspects.

The main challenge in the investigation of desvenlafaxine's role in migraine prophylaxis is the lack of official approval. As such, the derivation of clinically relevant data must be obtained from retrospective studies such as the current investigation, as well as from consensus and the personal experience of neurologists that used desvenlafaxine to control depressive symptoms in people with migraine. In general, the diagnosis of headache is challenging; for example, migraine symptoms could be mediated by the medication overuse headache (MOH) that could interfere with accurate migraine subtype diagnosis. MOH does not exclude a diagnosis of refractory migraine. The present study recruited data from females diagnosed with migraine. According to evidence, the risk of MOH is higher in females, especially those residing in developing countries or with low socioeconomic status [55–57]. MOH diagnosis can be easily confirmed by the withdrawal of medications leading to improvement in headache [58].

Another major clinical challenge in migraine assessment is the presence of comorbid pain conditions. According to one study, 51% of the patients with migraine reported having one or more comorbid painful conditions; this percentage rose to 70% in patients diagnosed with chronic migraine [59]. For example, fibromyalgia has been reported in around 30% of patients with migraine [59]. Furthermore, migraine is closely associated with psychological distress; one study underscored that depression, anxiety, and insomnia are among the non-painful conditions associated with migraine [60]. This could be an opportunity to use antidepressants such as desvenlafaxine to manage anxiety and depressive symptoms while keeping an eye on the possible improvement in migraine burden. Another challenge in migraine, besides the cultural and socioeconomic factors, is the educational competencies among healthcare practitioners in developing countries. Although headache symptoms are one of the most commonly reported in clinics, in some countries it is overlooked. This could be linked to the poor educational and professional services offered to these patients [61]. For example, in one study among neurology residents involving >200 participants, about 30% self-reported difficulties in diagnosing migraine, and the most reported barrier was the accurate communication and collaboration between the patient and the healthcare provider [62].

Our findings showed that desvenlafaxine was well-tolerated as only one case reported constipation at 100 mg dose, and this side effect subsided after dose reduction to 50 mg. This result is in line with the existing literature, which underscores the high tolerability profile of desvenlafaxine. However, dry mouth and constipation were reported in previous studies at the 50 mg and the 100 mg doses [63]. In addition, desvenlafaxine could be associated with vasoconstriction syndrome and severe headaches [64]. Besides its tolerability in general, desvenlafaxine's preferable pharmacokinetics, primarily its lower incidence of inhibiting the hepatic enzyme Cytochrome P450, which minimizes the chance of drug interactions, makes it an attractive choice for clinicians [38].

This work adds to the very little existing literature examining the role of desvenlafaxine in migraine prophylaxis, especially in women. However, the limited study sample prevents the generalization of the results. Therefore, future larger-scale follow-up studies are required to fully elucidate the potential efficacy of desvenlafaxine in migraine attack prevention. This is a small study using retrospective data. As such, the results are very preliminary. The study has a small sample size and is non-randomized. These are significant limitations for drawing general conclusions. Additionally, this was not a blinded and controlled trial. It did not rule out the placebo effect. It also did not rule out changes in migraine frequency. Larger, prospective, randomized controlled trials should address these limitations in the future. They could also investigate whether desvenlafaxine is effective for different types of migraine. They could also assess its long-term effectiveness and safety and could also compare it directly to other established prophylactic treatments. In short, this preliminary study analyzed data retrospectively from ten women with migraine using validated tools in its assessment and included clinical details of the patients' points facilitating the performance of larger-scale studies of the role of desvenlafaxine in migraine prophylaxis. The reported findings show an improvement in all the assessment parameters under investigation, namely, the number of migraine days per month, the average headache duration in minutes, the headache severity on the visual analog scale, and the frequency of acute medication use per week.

5. Conclusions

This study provides early preliminary evidence that supports the use of desvenlafaxine to prevent migraines in female patients. It may improve life quality and reduce the burden of migraines for patients. This fits with desvenlafaxine inhibiting both serotonin and norepinephrine reuptake. Desvenlafaxine was very well tolerated in our group. Only one case of mild side effects was noted. Although not conclusive, the results are promising. However, interpreters must approach the study's limitations with caution. The first limitation is its small sample size. The second is its retrospective nature. This work makes some discoveries. They add to very poor existing literature about desvenlafaxine in migraine prevention. They suggest it may be a valuable addition to the drugs for managing migraine, and that females with depression and migraine could benefit from desvenlafaxine. More research is required. It should be larger and prospective. The studies should be randomized and controlled. These studies need to fully demonstrate how well desvenlafaxine prevents migraines. They are also needed to show its place in clinical practice.

Author Contributions: Conceptualization, H.H.A.H., H.A.E.A. and O.G.; methodology, M.S.H., H.H.A.H. and M.R.; software, H.M.B., A.A.A.A. and Y.M.B.; validation, H.H.A.H., O.G. and M.S.H.; formal analysis O.G.; investigation, M.S.H. and M.R.; resources, H.H.A.H. and H.A.E.A.; data curation, H.A.E.A., Y.M.B. and H.M.B.; writing—original draft preparation, O.G. and A.A.A.A.; writing—review and editing, O.G., H.H.A.H. and A.A.A.A.; visualization, H.H.A.H.; M.R. supervision, O.G. and H.H.A.H.; project administration, H.A.E.A., H.M.B. and Y.M.B. funding acquisition, H.H.A.H. All authors have read and agreed to the published version of the manuscript.

Funding: This research was funded by United Pharmaceuticals Manufacturing Co., part of MS Pharma.

Institutional Review Board Statement: The study was conducted in accordance with the Declaration of Helsinki, and approved by the Institutional Review Board of Yarmouk University (protocol code (094/approved on 29 February 2024).

Informed Consent Statement: The clinicians obtained consent from the patients to use their data for scientific purposes, and all data were kept anonymous.

Data Availability Statement: All data related to this manuscript will be available from the corresponding author upon request.

Acknowledgments: The corresponding author would like to thank Sama, Suzi, Yasmina, and Nour. Also, special thanks to Nadera Najjar and Kefah Habash for their support.

Conflicts of Interest: The authors declare no conflicts of interest.

References

1. Lipton, R.B.; Bigal, M.E.; Diamond, M.; Freitag, F.; Reed, M.L.; Stewart, W.F. Migraine prevalence, disease burden, and the need for preventive therapy. *Neurology* **2007**, *68*, 343–349. [CrossRef] [PubMed]
2. Breslau, N.; Rasmussen, B.K. The impact of migraine: Epidemiology, risk factors, and co-morbidities. *Neurology* **2001**, *56* (Suppl. S1), S4–S12. [CrossRef] [PubMed]
3. Dahlöf, C.; Linde, M. One-year prevalence of migraine in Sweden: A population-based study in adults. *Cephalalgia* **2001**, *21*, 664–671. [CrossRef]
4. Lipton, R.B.; Stewart, W.F.; Diamond, S.; Diamond, M.L.; Reed, M. Prevalence and burden of migraine in the United States: Data from the American Migraine Study II. *Headache J. Head Face Pain* **2001**, *41*, 646–657. [CrossRef] [PubMed]
5. Moloney, M.F.; Matthews, K.B.; Scharbo-Dehaan, M.; Strickland, O.L. Caring for the woman with migraine headaches. *Nurse Pract.* **2000**, *25*, 17. [CrossRef]
6. Gibbs, T.S.; Fleischer, A.B., Jr.; Feldman, S.R.; Sam, M.C.; O'Donovan, C.A. Health care utilization in patients with migraine: Demographics and patterns of care in the ambulatory setting. *Headache J. Head Face Pain* **2003**, *43*, 330–335. [CrossRef]
7. Carleton, R.N.; Abrams, M.P.; Asmundson, G.J.G.; Antony, M.M.; McCabe, R.E. Pain-related anxiety and anxiety sensitivity across anxiety and depressive disorders. *J. Anxiety Disord.* **2009**, *23*, 791–798. [CrossRef]
8. Seddik, A.H.; Branner, J.C.; Ostwald, D.A.; Schramm, S.H.; Bierbaum, M.; Katsarava, Z. The socioeconomic burden of migraine: An evaluation of productivity losses due to migraine headaches based on a population study in Germany. *Cephalalgia* **2020**, *40*, 1551–1560. [CrossRef]
9. Feigin, V.L.; Abajobir, A.A.; Abate, K.H.; Abd-Allah, F.; Abdulle, A.M.; Abera, S.F.; Abyu, G.Y.; Ahmed, M.B.; Aichour, A.N.; Aichour, I.; et al. Global, regional, and national burden of neurological disorders during 1990–2015: A systematic analysis for the Global Burden of Disease Study 2015. *Lancet Neurol.* **2017**, *16*, 877–897. [CrossRef]
10. Steiner, T.J.; Stovner, L.J.; Jensen, R.; Uluduz, D.; Katsarava, Z.; Lifting The Burden: The Global Campaign against Headache. Migraine remains second among the world's causes of disability, and first among young women: Findings from GBD2019. *J. Headache Pain* **2020**, *21*, 137. [CrossRef]
11. Merikangas, K.R.; Risch, N.J.; Merikangas, J.R.; Weissman, M.M.; Kidd, K.K. Migraine and depression: Association and familial transmission. *J. Psychiatr. Res.* **1988**, *22*, 119–129. [CrossRef] [PubMed]
12. Breslau, N.; Schultz, L.R.; Stewart, W.F.; Lipton, R.B.; Lucia, V.C.; Welch, K.M.A. Headache and major depression: Is the association specific to migraine? *Neurology* **2000**, *54*, 308–313. [CrossRef] [PubMed]
13. Deen, M.; Christensen, C.E.; Hougaard, A.; Hansen, H.D.; Knudsen, G.M.; Ashina, M. Serotonergic mechanisms in the migraine brain—A systematic review. *Cephalalgia* **2017**, *37*, 251–264. [CrossRef] [PubMed]
14. Goadsby, P.J. Pathophysiology of migraine. *Neurol. Clin.* **2009**, *27*, 335–360. [CrossRef]
15. Noseda, R.; Burstein, R. Migraine pathophysiology: Anatomy of the trigeminovascular pathway and associated neurological symptoms, cortical spreading depression, sensitization, and modulation of pain. *Pain* **2013**, *154*, S44–S53. [CrossRef]
16. Jorgensen, H.S. Studies on the neuroendocrine role of serotonin. *Dan. Med. Bull.* **2007**, *54*, 266–288.
17. Celada, P.; Puig, M.V.; Artigas, F. Serotonin modulation of cortical neurons and networks. *Front. Integr. Neurosci.* **2013**, *7*, 25. [CrossRef]
18. Hornung, J.-P. The human raphe nuclei and the serotonergic system. *J. Chem. Neuroanat.* **2003**, *26*, 331–343. [CrossRef]
19. Ferrari, M.D.; Odink, J.; Tapparelli, C.; Van Kempen, G.M.J.; Pennings, E.J.M.; Bruyn, G.W. Serotonin metabolism in migraine. *Neurology* **1989**, *39*, 1239. [CrossRef]
20. Hamel, E.; Currents, H. Serotonin and migraine: Biology and clinical implications. *Cephalalgia* **2007**, *27*, 1293–1300. [CrossRef]
21. Obata, H. Analgesic mechanisms of antidepressants for neuropathic pain. *Int. J. Mol. Sci.* **2017**, *18*, 2483. [CrossRef] [PubMed]
22. Ossipov, M.H.; Dussor, G.O.; Porreca, F. Central modulation of pain. *J. Clin. Investig.* **2010**, *120*, 3779–3787. [CrossRef] [PubMed]
23. Pertovaara, A. The noradrenergic pain regulation system: A potential target for pain therapy. *Eur. J. Pharmacol.* **2013**, *716*, 2–7. [CrossRef] [PubMed]
24. Baron, R.; Binder, A.; Wasner, G. Neuropathic pain: Diagnosis, pathophysiological mechanisms, and treatment. *Lancet Neurol.* **2010**, *9*, 807–819. [CrossRef]
25. Zhou, M.; Gebhart, G.F. Inhibition of a cutaneous nociceptive reflex by a noxious visceral stimulus is mediated by spinal cholinergic and descending serotonergic systems in the rat. *Brain Res.* **1992**, *585*, 7–18. [CrossRef]
26. Holden, J.E.; Farah, E.N.; Jeong, Y. Stimulation of the lateral hypothalamus produces antinociception mediated by 5-HT1A, 5-HT1B and 5-HT3 receptors in the rat spinal cord dorsal horn. *Neuroscience* **2005**, *135*, 1255–1268. [CrossRef]
27. Blakely, R.D.; Bauman, A.L. Biogenic amine transporters: Regulation in flux. *Curr. Opin. Neurobiol.* **2000**, *10*, 328–336. [CrossRef]

28. Burgess, S.E.; Gardell, L.R.; Ossipov, M.H.; Malan, T.P.; Vanderah, T.W.; Lai, J.; Porreca, F. Time-dependent descending facilitation from the rostral ventromedial medulla maintains, but does not initiate, neuropathic pain. *J. Neurosci.* **2002**, *22*, 5129–5136. [CrossRef]
29. Young, W.B.; Bradley, K.C.; Anjum, M.W.; Gebeline-Myers, C. Duloxetine prophylaxis for episodic migraine in persons without depression: A prospective study. *Headache J. Head Face Pain* **2013**, *53*, 1430–1437. [CrossRef]
30. Wang, F.; Wang, J.; Cao, Y.; Xu, Z. Serotonin-norepinephrine reuptake inhibitors for the prevention of migraine and vestibular migraine: A systematic review and meta-analysis. *Reg. Anesth. Pain Med.* **2020**, *45*, 323–330. [CrossRef]
31. Marks, D.M.; Shah, M.J.; Patkar, A.A.; Masand, P.S.; Park, G.-Y.; Pae, C.-U. Serotonin-norepinephrine reuptake inhibitors for pain control: Premise and promise. *Curr. Neuropharmacol.* **2009**, *7*, 331–336. [CrossRef] [PubMed]
32. Robinson, C.; Dalal, S.; Chitneni, A.; Patil, A.; Berger, A.A.; Mahmood, S.; Orhurhu, V.; Kaye, A.D.; Hasoon, J. A look at commonly utilized serotonin noradrenaline reuptake inhibitors (SNRIs) in chronic pain. *Health Psychol. Res.* **2022**, *10*, 32309. [CrossRef] [PubMed]
33. Pringsheim, T.; Davenport, W.J.; Becker, W.J. Prophylaxis of migraine headache. *CMAJ* **2010**, *182*, E269–E276. [CrossRef]
34. Bulut, S.; Berilgen, M.S.; Baran, A.; Tekatas, A.; Atmaca, M.; Mungen, B. Venlafaxine versus amitriptyline in the prophylactic treatment of migraine: Randomized, double-blind, crossover study. *Clin. Neurol. Neurosurg.* **2004**, *107*, 44–48. [CrossRef] [PubMed]
35. Raffaelli, B.; Reuter, U. The biology of monoclonal antibodies: Focus on calcitonin gene-related peptide for prophylactic migraine therapy. *Neurotherapeutics* **2018**, *15*, 324–335. [CrossRef]
36. Silberstein, S.D. Practice parameter: Evidence-based guidelines for migraine headache (an evidence-based review) [RETIRED] Report of the Quality Standards Subcommittee of the American Academy of Neurology. *Neurology* **2000**, *55*, 754–762. [CrossRef]
37. Boyer, P.; Montgomery, S.; Lepola, U.; Germain, J.-M.; Brisard, C.; Ganguly, R.; Padmanabhan, S.K.; Tourian, K.A. Efficacy, safety, and tolerability of fixed-dose desvenlafaxine 50 and 100 mg/day for major depressive disorder in a placebo-controlled trial. *Int. Clin. Psychopharmacol.* **2008**, *23*, 243–253. [CrossRef]
38. Oganesian, A.; Shilling, A.D.; Young-Sciame, R.; Tran, J.; Watanyar, A.; Azam, F.; Kao, J.; Leung, L. Desvenlafaxine and venlafaxine exert minimal in vitro inhibition of human cytochrome P450 and P-glycoprotein activities. *Psychopharmacol. Bull.* **2009**, *42*, 47–63.
39. Allen, R.; Sharma, U.; Barlas, S. Clinical experience with desvenlafaxine in treatment of pain associated with diabetic peripheral neuropathy. *J. Pain Res.* **2014**, *7*, 339–351. [CrossRef]
40. Goswami, M.; Mahanta, A.; Yanamandra, V.; Das, M. Migraine Prophylaxis—A study of effectiveness and side effects of various drugs used in migraine prophylaxis. *Eur. J. Cardiovasc. Med.* **2024**, *14*, 74–79.
41. Bonilla-Jaime, H.; Sánchez-Salcedo, J.A.; Estevez-Cabrera, M.M.; Molina-Jiménez, T.; Cortes-Altamirano, J.L.; Alfaro-Rodríguez, A. Depression and pain: Use of antidepressants. *Curr. Neuropharmacol.* **2022**, *20*, 384. [CrossRef] [PubMed]
42. Diamond, M. The impact of migraine on the health and well-being of women. *J. Women's Health* **2007**, *16*, 1269–1280. [CrossRef] [PubMed]
43. D'Amico, D.; Tepper, S.J. Prophylaxis of migraine: General principles and patient acceptance. *Neuropsychiatr. Dis. Treat.* **2008**, *4*, 1155–1167. [CrossRef] [PubMed]
44. Dowson, A.J.; Massiou, H.; Aurora, S.K. Managing migraine headaches experienced by patients who self–report with menstrually related migraine: A prospective, placebo–controlled study with oral sumatriptan. *J. Headache Pain* **2005**, *6*, 81–87. [CrossRef] [PubMed]
45. Galer, B.S. Neuropathic pain of peripheral origin: Advances in pharmacologic treatment. *Neurology* **1995**, *45* (Suppl. S9), S17–S25. [CrossRef] [PubMed]
46. Dwight, M.M.; Arnold, L.M.; O'brien, H.; Metzger, R.; Morris-Park, E.; Keck, P.E., Jr. An open clinical trial of venlafaxine treatment of fibromyalgia. *Psychosomatics* **1998**, *39*, 14–17. [CrossRef] [PubMed]
47. Taylor, K.; Rowbotham, M.C. Venlafaxine hydrochloride and chronic pain. *West. J. Med.* **1996**, *165*, 147.
48. Couch, J.R.; Hassanein, R.S. Amitriptyline in migraine prophylaxis. *Arch. Neurol.* **1979**, *36*, 695–699. [CrossRef]
49. Gomersall, J.D.; Stuart, A. Amitriptyline in migraine prophylaxis: Changes in pattern of attacks during a controlled clinical trial. *J. Neurol. Neurosurg. Psychiatry* **1973**, *36*, 684–690. [CrossRef]
50. Schweizer, E.; Thielen, R.J.; Frazer, A. Venlafaxine: A novel antidepressant compound. *Expert Opin. Investig. Drugs* **1997**, *6*, 65–78. [CrossRef]
51. Bryant, S.G.; Pharmd; Fisher, S.; Kluge, R.M. Long-term versus short-term amitriptyline side effects as measured by a postmarketing surveillance system. *J. Clin. Psychopharmacol.* **1987**, *7*, 78–82. [CrossRef] [PubMed]
52. Dierick, M. A review of the efficacy and tolerability of venlafaxine. *Eur. Psychiatry* **1997**, *12*, 307s–313s. [CrossRef] [PubMed]
53. Adelman, L.C.; Adelman, J.U.; Von Seggern, R.; Mannix, L.K. Venlafaxine extended release (XR) for the prophylaxis of migraine and tension-type headache: A retrospective study in a clinical setting. *Headache* **2000**, *40*, 572–580. [CrossRef] [PubMed]
54. Ozyalcin, S.N.; Talu, G.K.; Kiziltan, E.; Yucel, B.; Ertas, M.; Disci, R. The efficacy and safety of venlafaxine in the prophylaxis of migraine. *Headache* **2005**, *45*, 144–152. [CrossRef]
55. González-Oria, C.; Belvís, R.; Cuadrado, M.; Díaz-Insa, S.; Guerrero-Peral, A.; Huerta, M.; Irimia, P.; Láinez, J.; Latorre, G.; Leira, R.; et al. Document of revision and updating of medication overuse headache (MOH). *Neurol. (Engl. Ed.)* **2021**, *36*, 229–240. [CrossRef]

56. Laskar, S.; Kalita, J.; Misra, U.K. Comparison of chronic daily headache with and without medication overuse headache using ICHD II R and ICHD 3 beta criteria. *Clin. Neurol. Neurosurg.* **2019**, *183*, 105382. [CrossRef]
57. Robblee, J. Breaking the cycle: Unraveling the diagnostic, pathophysiological and treatment challenges of refractory migraine. *Front. Neurol.* **2023**, *14*, 1263535. [CrossRef]
58. Robbins, M.S. Diagnosis and management of headache: A review. *JAMA* **2021**, *325*, 1874–1885. [CrossRef]
59. Henningsen, P.; Hausteiner-Wiehle, C.; Häuser, W. Migraine in the context of chronic primary pain, chronic overlapping pain disorders, and functional somatic disorders: A narrative review. *Headache J. Head Face Pain* **2022**, *62*, 1272–1280. [CrossRef]
60. Buse, D.; Manack, A.; Serrano, D.; Reed, M.; Varon, S.; Turkel, C.; Lipton, R. Headache impact of chronic and episodic migraine: Results from the American Migraine Prevalence and Prevention study. *Headache J. Head Face Pain* **2012**, *52*, 3–17. [CrossRef]
61. Martelletti, P.; Steiner, T. Headache disorders: Building specialist education. In *Headache Care, Research and Education Worldwide*, 17th ed.; Oxford University Press: Oxford, UK, 2010; pp. 173–178.
62. Tawakul, A.A.; Aldharman, S.S.; Al-Rabiah, N.M.; Alqarni, G.S.; Albalawi, A.A.; Alhussaini, O.M.; Alhazmi, N.F.; Alharbi, A.R.; Babateen, O.; Tawakul, A.A.; et al. Assessment of Barriers and Challenges in Headache Education among Neurology Residents in Saudi Arabia. *Cureus* **2023**, *15*, e38328. [CrossRef] [PubMed]
63. Liebowitz, M.R.; Manley, A.L.; Padmanabhan, S.K.; Ganguly, R.; Tummala, R.; Tourian, K.A. Efficacy, safety, and tolerability of desvenlafaxine 50 mg/day and 100 mg/day in outpatients with major depressive disorder. *Curr. Med. Res. Opin.* **2008**, *24*, 1877–1890. [CrossRef] [PubMed]
64. Abu-Abaa, M.; AbuBakar, M.; Mousa, A.; Landau, D. Desvenlafaxine As the Main Possible Culprit in Triggering Reversible Cerebral Vasoconstriction Syndrome: A Case Report. *Cureus* **2022**, *14*, e29780. [CrossRef] [PubMed]

Disclaimer/Publisher's Note: The statements, opinions and data contained in all publications are solely those of the individual author(s) and contributor(s) and not of MDPI and/or the editor(s). MDPI and/or the editor(s) disclaim responsibility for any injury to people or property resulting from any ideas, methods, instructions or products referred to in the content.

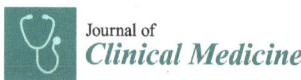
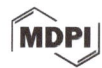

Systematic Review

Safety and Efficacy of Atogepant for the Preventive Treatment of Migraines in Adults: A Systematic Review and Meta-Analysis

Abdulrahim Saleh Alrasheed [1,*], Taif Mansour Almaqboul [2], Reem Ali Alshamrani [3], Noor Mohammad AlMohish [4] and Majed Mohammad Alabdali [5]

- [1] College of Medicine, King Faisal University, AlAhsa 31982, Saudi Arabia
- [2] College of Medicine, Batterjee Medical College, Jeddah 21442, Saudi Arabia; 150341.taif@bmc.edu.sa
- [3] College of Medicine, Taif University, Taif 21944, Saudi Arabia; reemalshamrani-@hotmail.com
- [4] Neurology Department, King Fahad Hospital of the University, Imam Abdulrahman Bin Faisal University, Khobar 34445, Saudi Arabia; nmalmohish@iau.edu.sa
- [5] Neurology Department, College of Medicine, Imam Abdulrahman Bin Faisal University, Khobar 34445, Saudi Arabia; mmalabdali@iau.edu.sa
- * Correspondence: 221414880@student.kfu.edu.sa or abdulrhim2003@hotmail.com

Abstract: Background: Migraine is a common neurological condition marked by unilateral recurrent pulsating headaches, often associated with systemic signs and symptoms. Recently, calcitonin gene-related peptide (CGRP) antagonists, including atogepant, an oral CGRP receptor antagonist, have emerged as effective and safe treatments. The current study sought to assess the efficacy and safety of atogepant for preventing episodic migraines in adults. **Methods:** A comprehensive search, following PRISMA guidelines, was conducted using PubMed, Web of Science, and Cochrane Library to identify randomized, double-blind, placebo-controlled trials published up to June 2024. **Results:** The studies included adult participants with episodic migraine treated with atogepant. The primary outcomes assessed were changes in mean monthly migraine days (MMDs) and monthly headache days (MHDs) over 12 weeks. Secondary outcomes included reduction in acute medication use, 50% responder rates, and adverse events. A meta-analysis using a random-effects model was performed to evaluate efficacy and safety. Six trials with 4569 participants were included. Atogepant significantly reduced mean monthly migraine days (MMDs) and monthly headache days (MHDs) compared to placebo at all doses (10 mg, 30 mg, 60 mg), with the 60 mg dose showing the greatest reduction (mean difference: −1.48 days, $p < 0.001$). Significant reductions in acute medication use and improved 50% responder rates were also observed for all doses. The safety profile of atogepant was favorable, with common adverse events being mild to moderate, such as constipation and nausea. There were no significant differences in serious adverse events between the atogepant and placebo groups. **Conclusions:** Atogepant is an effective and well-tolerated option for preventing episodic migraines, showing significant reductions in migraine frequency and acute medication use. However, further studies are necessary to assess its long-term safety and efficacy, especially at higher doses, and to investigate its potential role in personalized treatment strategies for migraine prevention.

Keywords: atogepant; CGRP receptor antagonist; preventive treatment; episodic migraine

1. Introduction

Migraine is a prevalent and debilitating neurological condition marked by unilateral recurrent pulsating moderate to severe attacks of headache, often associated with systemic symptoms such as vomiting, nausea, and sensitivity to sound and light [1]. It affects approximately 12% of the global population, with a higher incidence in women compared to men [2,3]. Migraines disproportionately affect individuals during their most productive years, typically between the ages of 18 and 44 [3]. The recurrent nature of migraines leads to frequent absenteeism and presenteeism, severely impacting professional and academic performance [4]. Moreover, the unpredictable onset of migraines contributes to anxiety and depression [5]. Migraine significantly impacts quality of life, leading to substantial personal, social, and economic burdens [6].

Migraine can be classified into two major types according to the International Classification of Headache Disorders (ICHD-3): episodic and chronic. The episodic form is characterized by headache attacks occurring on less than 15 days per month, whereas the chronic form involves headaches on 15 or more days per month, persisting for more than 3 months, with the diagnostic criteria including at least 8 days per month of migraine headaches. The distinction between these types is important for treatment and management strategies [7].

Treatment for migraine includes both acute and preventive approaches [8]. Acute treatments, which include triptans, non-steroidal anti-inflammatory drugs (NSAIDs), and antiemetics, are intended to relieve symptoms during an attack. Preventive treatments, including botulinum toxin A, antidepressants, anticonvulsants, and antihypertensive drugs, are used to lower the incidence, severity, and duration of migraines, thereby improving the overall quality of life for sufferers [8,9]. Approximately 50–60% of patients benefit from preventive treatments, highlighting their importance in migraine management [10,11]. However, these were traditional treatments for migraine, and they are non-specific migraine treatments with limited degrees of effectiveness, prompting the need for more effective and tolerable therapeutic options [12,13].

The advent of calcitonin gene-related peptide (CGRP) receptor antagonists represents a significant advancement in the management of migraine [14]. CGRP plays a crucial role in migraine pathophysiology by modulating pain pathways and vascular functions. CGRP is released during migraine attacks and contributes to the inflammation and dilation of cerebral blood vessels. The development of CGRP antagonists offers a targeted approach to migraine treatment, providing relief with fewer side effects compared to traditional therapies [15].

For the prevention of migraine, there are several monoclonal antibodies acting on the CGRP pathway; erenumab targets the CGRP receptor, while eptinezumab, fremanezumab, and galcanezumab block the CGRP ligand. Rimegepant and ubrogepant, two oral CGRP receptor antagonists, are licensed for the management of migraine attacks. Rimegepant also gained approval for the prevention of migraines in adults in 2021, making it the only medication that may be used for both acute and preventive treatment of migraines [16]. Although these monoclonal antibodies (MAbs) have been used for the prevention of migraine attacks, patients experienced some discomfort from the subcutaneous or intravenous delivery of these medications [12]. In contrast to preventive monoclonal antibodies, CGRP receptor antagonists (gepants), are primarily administered as pills, nasal sprays, and orally disintegrating tablets (ODT) [17].

Atogepant stands out as one of the oral drugs established for the preventive treatment of episodic migraine. It was accepted by the FDA on 15 September 2021, and is available in doses of 10 mg, 30 mg, and 60 mg [9].

Approximated to additional CGRP receptor antagonists like rimegepant, atogepant, an oral CGRP receptor antagonist authorized for the preventive treatment of episodic migraine, has several significant benefits [18,19]. Rimegepant is certified for both acute and preventive therapy; however, because it is dosed every other day for prevention, adherence issues may arise. Contrarily, atogepant is only meant to be taken once daily, making it easier to follow and more convenient for patients [19]. Furthermore, atogepant has a well-established track record of lowering monthly migraine days (MMDs), with notable reductions in MMDs and a positive safety record. This once-a-day oral medication provides an opportune, secure, and efficient preventive outcome [18]. It is especially appropriate for individuals who would choose a daily dosage regimen without the intrusiveness of injectables [19]. The current study sought to assess the efficacy and safety of atogepant for preventing episodic migraines in adults.

2. Methods

This systematic review and meta-analysis adhered to the Preferred Reporting Items for Systematic Reviews and Meta-Analyses (PRISMA) guidelines. Prospectively, we registered the study protocol in the International Prospective Register of Systematic Reviews (PROSPERO) (registration number: CRD42024556275).

2.1. Search Strategy

We systematically searched the PubMed, Cochrane Library, and Web of Science databases through June 2024. The search strategy used a combination of Medical Subject Headings (MeSH) and the following Boolean operators: "Migraine" OR "Episodic Migraine" OR "Recurrent Migraine" OR "Refractory Migraine" OR "Headache" OR "Recurrent Headache" OR "Refractory Headache" AND "Efficacy" OR "Safety" OR "Tolerability" OR "Outcome" OR "Findings" OR "Impact" AND "Atogepant" OR "Preventive Treatment" OR "Preventive Therapy" OR "Prevention" AND "Random" OR "Placebo" OR "Trial" OR "Group". The retrieved study reference lists were revised to identify other relevant articles.

2.2. Eligibility Criteria

The studies included in this review were randomized, placebo-controlled trials involving participants aged ≥18 years with a history of migraine for at least twelve months, with onset before age 50. Participants needed to experience 4–14 monthly migraine days (MMDs) during the three months prior to screening and record this data in an electronic diary during a 28-day baseline period. Only English-language papers were considered. Exclusion criteria included studies that did not report outcomes of interest, review articles, and case reports.

2.3. Outcome Measures

The evaluated primary efficacy outcomes included changes from baseline in the mean number of monthly migraine days (MMDs), monthly headache days (MHDs), and the number of acute-medications-use days per month. Additionally, the percentage of participants who experienced at least a 50% reduction in migraine days per month during the double-blind treatment phase was assessed.

Secondary efficacy outcomes involved evaluating changes from baseline in the average number of acute-medications-use days. Safety and tolerability outcomes included rates of adverse events (AEs), withdrawals due to AEs, and serious adverse events (SAEs). Key safety measures were treatment emergent adverse events (TEAEs).

2.4. Study Selection, Data Extraction, and Quality Assessment

We used Rayyan Software (Version 1.5.0, Qatar Computing Research Institute, Doha, Qatar) to manage electronic database search results for selection, screening, and duplicate removal. Titles and abstracts were screened by two independent reviewers, with any disagreements resolved by involving a third reviewer.

Data extraction was conducted by two independent reviewers, focusing on study characteristics, participant demographics, intervention specifics, and outcomes. Any disagreements were resolved through discussion. Extracted data included author details, publication year, journal name, country, study design, and key trial elements such as randomization, blinding, treatment periods, and atogepant doses (10, 30, and 60 mg once daily). Screening, randomization, and follow-up periods were noted, alongside inclusion and exclusion criteria. Participant demographics covered age, gender, race, and ethnicity. Outcome measures, along with the total number of participants, group distributions, analysis populations, and safety metrics, were documented.

The risk of bias was independently assessed by two reviewers using the Cochrane Risk of Bias 2 (RoB 2) tool via Review Manager 5.4 software (The Cochrane Collaboration, London, UK), with any disagreements resolved through discussion or consultation with a third reviewer [20,21]. The quality assessment of the included studies was conducted utilizing the Revised Cochrane Risk of Bias Assessment Tool 2. The evidence certainty for each outcome was evaluated using the GRADE approach, which considered factors such as the robustness of the data, potential selective reporting, and other bias sources. Evidence was downgraded for serious or very serious concerns [22].

2.5. Statistical Analysis

Heterogeneity among the trials was evaluated by the funnel plot visual examination, the chi-squared test, and I^2 statistics. A fixed-effect model was planned for use when heterogeneity was not significant ($p > 0.05$) [23,24]. However, the decision between a fixed-effect or random-effects model was primarily based on the I^2 value: a fixed-effect model was planned to be applied when I^2 was less than 40%, while a random-effects model was utilized for I^2 values of 40% or greater. The measures of association between treatment and continuous or dichotomous outcomes were the mean difference (MD) and risk ratio (RR), both reported alongside 95% confidence intervals (CIs).

During the double-blind treatment period, all efficacy analyses were carried out on the modified intention-to-treat population, encompassing all randomly allocated participants who had a minimum of one dose of atogepant, assessable baseline electronic recorded data, and a minimum of one evaluable post-baseline 4-week period of electronic recorded diary. All individuals who received at least one dosage of the study drug were included in the safety and tolerability evaluations. Two-sided p-values were reported, and $p < 0.05$ was considered significant. The data were analyzed using Review Manager software version 5.4.

3. Results

3.1. Search Results

A flowchart illustrating the study selection process is shown in (Figure 1). Our search identified 71 records. These included 35 duplicate articles that were removed, leaving 36 unique articles for screening by title and abstract. Out of the 36 articles screened, 18 were excluded as they did not meet the eligibility criteria. The remaining 18 full-text articles were reviewed for more detailed evaluation and 12 articles were excluded because 9 of them did not report on relevant episodic migraine preventive therapy and three articles did not report the outcomes of interest. Finally, six studies were included in our study [9,11,25–28].

3.2. Quality Assessment

In the risk-of-bias assessment, three of the six included studies exhibited potential concerns. Specifically, issues related to randomization and missing outcome data were identified in two trials [9,25]. In contrast, the remaining three studies [11,26,28] were determined to have a minimal risk of bias (Figure 2).

3.3. Characteristics of the Included Studies

The current review included six studies, where a total of 1231 participants were allocated randomly to placebo, 977 to atogepant 10 mg, 1095 to atogepant 30 mg, and 1266 to atogepant 60 mg, for a total of 4569 participants [9,11,25–28]. Participants' ages ranged from 18 to 73 years; 87.2% were females, 12.8% were males, and 81.9% were white. However, no data were provided about the patients' ethnic origin in any of the studied articles. The mean BMI ranged from 26.2 (5.2) in Tassorelli et al.'s 2024 [28] study to 31.1 ± 7.6 kg/m^2 in Ailani et al.'s 2021 [11] study. Among studies that provided relevant data, 97.8% of the participants reported current use of acute medications. In terms of migraine frequency, the monthly migraine days (MMD) during the 28-day baseline period ranged from 7 to 14 days. Notably, only Goadsby et al., 2020 [26] assessed the migraine associated with aura, where 21.5% of the participants reported such association. Baseline monthly headache days (MHD) were assessed in four articles [11,25–27] and were found to range from 4 to 14 days. Furthermore, only two studies [25,27] assessed the baseline monthly acute-medications-use days, reporting a mean of 6.5 to 6.9 days (Table 1).

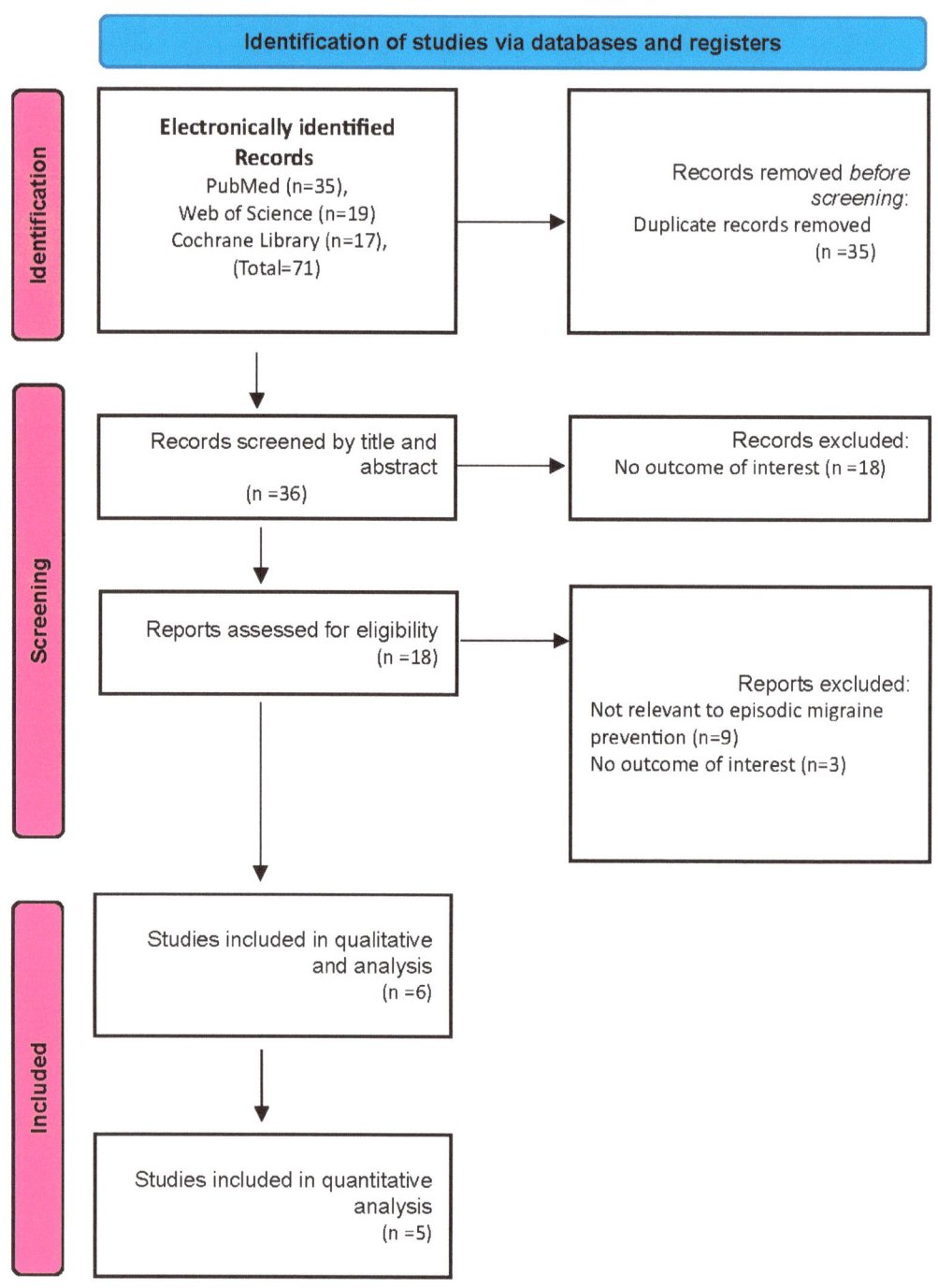

Figure 1. PRISMA flowchart.

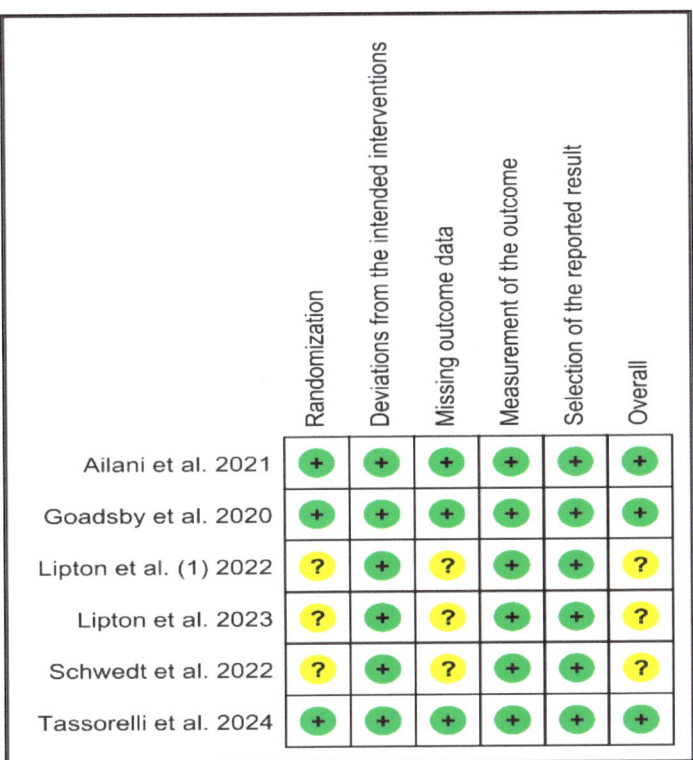

Figure 2. Quality assessment of the included studies [9,11,25–28].

3.4. Meta-Analysis

The forest plots and meta-analysis were performed using Review Manager software version 5.4. All results were subjected to a random-effects model. Mean differences (MD) were utilized to report continuous outcomes, while risk ratios (RR) were used to represent dichotomous outcomes. Publication bias was visually assessed using a funnel plot, and heterogeneity was quantified using the I^2 statistic and the Chi^2 test p-value. A 95% confidence interval was applied to all estimates, and results were considered statistically significant if the p-value was less than 0.05.

3.5. Mean Monthly Migraine Days Change from Baseline

Three studies were included in the analysis, revealing that atogepant significantly outperformed placebo in reducing mean monthly migraine days across various subgroups. The observed mean differences were as follows: −1.16 days for atogepant 10 mg ($p < 0.001$, $I^2 = 0\%$), −1.15 days for atogepant 30 mg ($p < 0.001$, $I^2 = 36\%$), and −1.48 days for atogepant 60 mg ($p = 0.0009$, $I^2 = 79\%$). While no significant heterogeneity was detected in the atogepant 10 mg and 30 mg subgroups, a substantial degree of heterogeneity was present in the atogepant 60 mg subgroup, attributed to random error. The p-value for the atogepant 60 mg subgroup was 0.0009, with an I^2 of 79%. Although the study by Schwedt et al. (2022) was excluded from this analysis due to missing data, its findings align with those of the included studies. Schwedt et al. (2022) reported that atogepant significantly reduced the mean monthly migraine days from baseline across all dosages (10 mg, 30 mg, and 60 mg) over all follow-up periods (1–4 weeks, 5–8 weeks, and 9–12 weeks) [25] (Figure 3).

Table 1. Baseline characteristics of the Included Studies.

	Goadsby et al., 2020 [26]				Schwedt et al., 2022 [25]			
Variable	Placebo	Atogepant 10 mg Once Daily	Atogepant 30 mg Once Daily	Atogepant 60 mg Once Daily	Placebo	Atogepant 10 mg Once Daily	Atogepant 30 mg Once Daily	Atogepant 60 mg Once Daily
Total sample size	186	93	183	186	222	221	228	231
Modified intention to treat population	178	92	182	177	214	214	223	222
Age, years	40.5 (11.7)	39.4 (12.4)	41.0 (13.6)	40.4 (11.7)	40.3 (12.8)	41.4 (12.1)	42.1 (11.7)	42.5 (12.4)
Female sex	154 (83%)	82 (88%)	166 (91%)	156 (84%)	198 (89.2%)	200 (90.5%)	204 (89.5%)	199 (86.1%)
White race	137 (74%)	69 (74%)	145 (79%)	133 (72%)	194 (87.4%)	181 (81.9%)	185 (81.1%)	192 (83.1%)
Black race	45 (24%)	20 (22%)	29 (16%)	44 (24%)	N/A	N/A	N/A	N/A
Other races	4 (2%)	4 (4%)	9 (5%)	9 (5%)	199 (89.6%)	200 (90.5%)	209 (91.7%)	217 (93.9%)
Body mass index, kg/m	30.4 (7.6)	29.9 (7.3)	30.0 (7.1)	30.0 (7.8)	30.8 (8.7)	30.4 (7.6)	31.2 (7.6)	29.9 (7.3)
Monthly migraine days	7.8 (2.5)	7.6 (2.5)	7.6 (2.4)	7.7 (2.6)	7.5 (2.4)	7.5 (2.5)	7.9 (2.3)	7.8 (2.3)
Migraine with aura	45 (24%)	21 (23%)	37 (20%)	36 (19%)	N/A	N/A	N/A	N/A
Migraine without aura	94 (51%)	48 (52%)	93 (51%)	96 (52%)	N/A	N/A	N/A	N/A
Monthly headache days	9.1 (2.7)	8.9 (2.7)	8.7 (2.5)	8.9 (2.8)	8.4 (2.6)	8.4 (2.8)	8.8 (2.6)	9.0 (2.6)
Monthly acute medication use days	6.6 (3.2)	6.2 (3.3)	6.6 (3.0)	6.8 (3.3)	6.5 (3.2)	6.6 (3.0)	6.7 (3.0)	6.9 (3.2)

	Tassorelli et al., 2024 [28]				Ailani et al., 2021 [11]			
Variable	Placebo	Atogepant 10 mg Once Daily	Atogepant 30 mg Once Daily	Atogepant 60 mg Once Daily	Placebo	Atogepant 10 mg Once Daily	Atogepant 30 mg Once Daily	Atogepant 60 mg Once Daily
Total sample size	157	N/A	N/A	156	222	221	228	231
Modified intention to treat population	154	N/A	N/A	151	214	214	223	222
Age, years	43.4 (10.3)	N/A	N/A	40.9 (10.7)	40.3 (12.8)	41.4 (12.0)	42.1 (11.7)	42.5 (12.4)
Female sex	141 (90%)	N/A	N/A	139 (89%)	198 (89.2%)	200 (90.5%)	204 (89.5%)	199 (86.1%)
White race	151 (96%)	N/A	N/A	149 (96%)	194 (87.4%)	181 (81.9%)	185 (81.1%)	192 (83.1%)
Black race	4 (3%)	N/A	N/A	3 (2%)	24 (10.8%)	34 (15.4%)	38 (16.7%)	28 (12.1%)
Other races	2 (1%)	N/A	N/A	2 (1%)	4 (1.8%)	6 (2.8%)	5 (2.1%)	10 (4.3%)
Body mass index, kg/m	26.2 (5.2)	N/A	N/A	25.6 (4.9)	30.8 (8.7)	30.3 (7.6)	31.1 (7.6)	29.9 (7.3)
Monthly migraine days	N/A	N/A	N/A	N/A	7.7 (2.6)	7.2 (2.5)	7.3 (2.4)	7.3 (2.4)
Migraine with aura	N/A	N/A	N/A	N/A	N/A	N/A	N/A	N/A
Migraine without aura	N/A	N/A	N/A	N/A	N/A	N/A	N/A	N/A
Monthly headache days	9.1 (2.7)	N/A	N/A	N/A	9.5 (2.8)	9.3 (2.7)	9.2 (2.7)	9.1 (2.7)
Monthly acute medication use days	N/A	N/A	N/A	N/A	N/A	N/A	N/A	N/A

Table 1. *Cont.*

	Lipton et al., 2023 [27]				Lipton et al., 2022 [9]			
Variable	Placebo	Atogepant 10 mg Once Daily	Atogepant 30 mg Once Daily	Atogepant 60 mg Once Daily	Placebo	Atogepant 10 mg Once Daily	Atogepant 30 mg Once Daily	Atogepant 60 mg Once Daily
Total sample size	222	221	228	231	222	221	228	231
Modified intention to treat population	214	214	223	222	214	214	223	222
Age, years	40.3 (12.9)	41.5 (12.0)	42.2 (11.7)	42.8 (12.3)	40.3 (12.8)	41.4 (12.1)	42.1 (11.7)	42.5 (12.4)
Female sex	190 (88.8%)	193 (90.2%)	199 (89.2%)	191 (86.0%)	198 (89.2%)	200 (90.5%)	204 (89.5%)	199 (86.1%)
White race	188 (87.9%)	176 (82.2%)	181 (81.2%)	184 (82.9%)	194 (87.4%)	181 (81.9%)	185 (81.1%)	192 (83.1%)
Black race	22 (10.3%)	32 (15.0%)	37 (16.6%)	27 (12.2%)	24 (10.8%)	34 (15.4%)	38 (16.7%)	28 (12.1%)
Other races	4 (1.8%)	6 (2.8%)	5 (2.2%)	11 (5%)	4 (1.8%)	6 (2.8%)	5 (2.1%)	11 (4.7%)
Body mass index, kg/m	N/A	N/A	N/A	N/A	30.8 (8.7%)	30.4 (7.6%)	31.2 (7.6%)	29.9 (7.3%)
Monthly migraine days baseline	7.5 (2.4)	7.5 (2.5)	7.9 (2.3)	7.8 (2.3)	7.5 (2.4)	7.5 (2.5)	7.9 (2.3)	7.8 (2.3)
Migraine with aura	N/A	N/A	N/A	N/A	N/A	N/A	N/A	N/A
Migraine without aura	N/A	N/A	N/A	N/A	N/A	N/A	N/A	N/A
Monthly headache days	8.4 (2.6)	8.4 (2.8)	8.8 (2.6)	9.0 (2.6)	N/A	N/A	N/A	N/A
Monthly acute medication use days	6.5 (3.2)	6.6 (3.0)	6.7 (3.0)	6.9 (3.2)	N/A	N/A	N/A	N/A

Data are reported as: N (%) or mean (SD); N/A: not applicable.

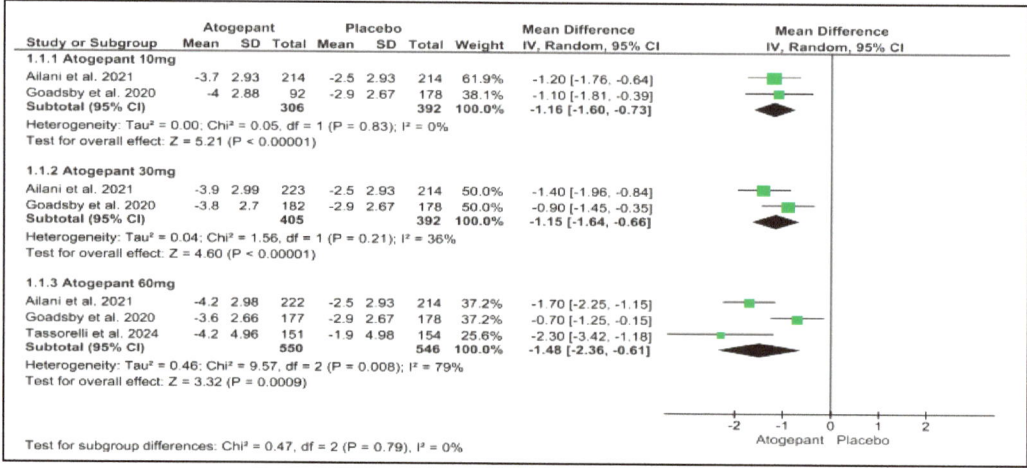

Figure 3. Mean monthly migraine days change from baseline forest plot [11,26,28].

3.6. Mean Monthly Headache Days Change from Baseline

This analysis included three trials, each of which indicated a substantial reduction in mean monthly headache days from baseline throughout a 12-week follow-up period for all atogepant dosages. None of the subgroups exhibited any detectable heterogeneity. Monthly headache days were reduced by 1.40 days for atogepant 10 mg ($p < 0.001$, $I^2 = 0\%$), −1.44 days for atogepant 30 mg ($p < 0.001$, $I^2 = 0\%$), and −1.63 days for atogepant 60 mg ($p < 0.001$, $I^2 = 49\%$). Furthermore, the study conducted by Schwedt et al. (2022) confirms the efficacy of atogepant (10 mg, 30 mg, and 60 mg) in dramatically lowering the mean number of monthly headache days from baseline over a 4-week period [25] (Figure 4).

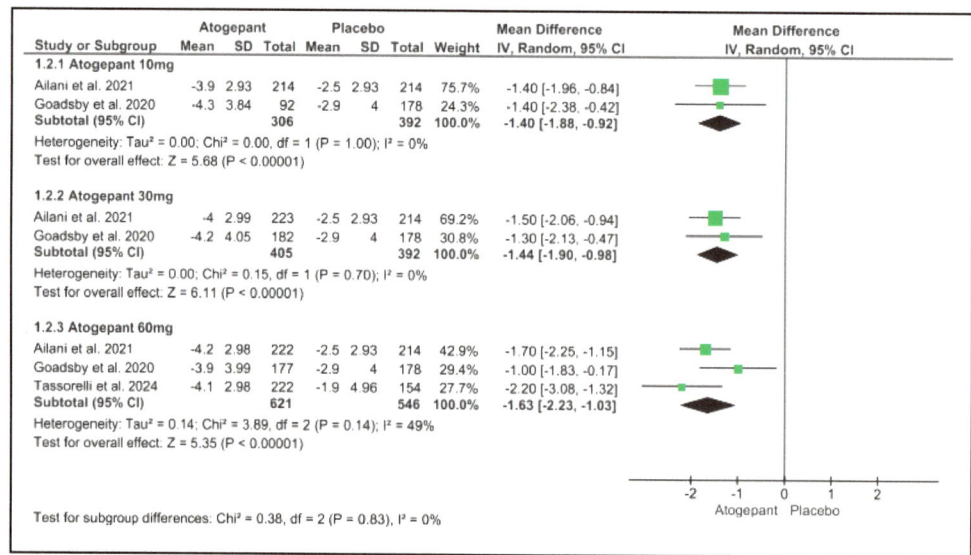

Figure 4. Mean monthly headache days change from baseline forest plot [11,26,28].

3.7. Acute Medication Use Days Change from Baseline

Over the 12-week follow-up period, atogepant (10 mg, 30 mg, and 60 mg) significantly reduced the requirement for acute medicines. There was no noticeable heterogeneity among the subgroups. Atogepant's mean differences at 10 mg, 30 mg, and 60 mg were -1.30, -1.40, and less than 0.001, $I^2 = 0\%$, and -1.58, with a p-value less than 0.001 and $I^2 = 65\%$, respectively. Schwedt et al. (2022) found that atogepant considerably reduced the requirement for acute treatment at all doses (10 mg, 30 mg, and 60 mg) and follow-up intervals (1–4 weeks, 5–8 weeks, and 9–12 weeks [25] (Figure 5).

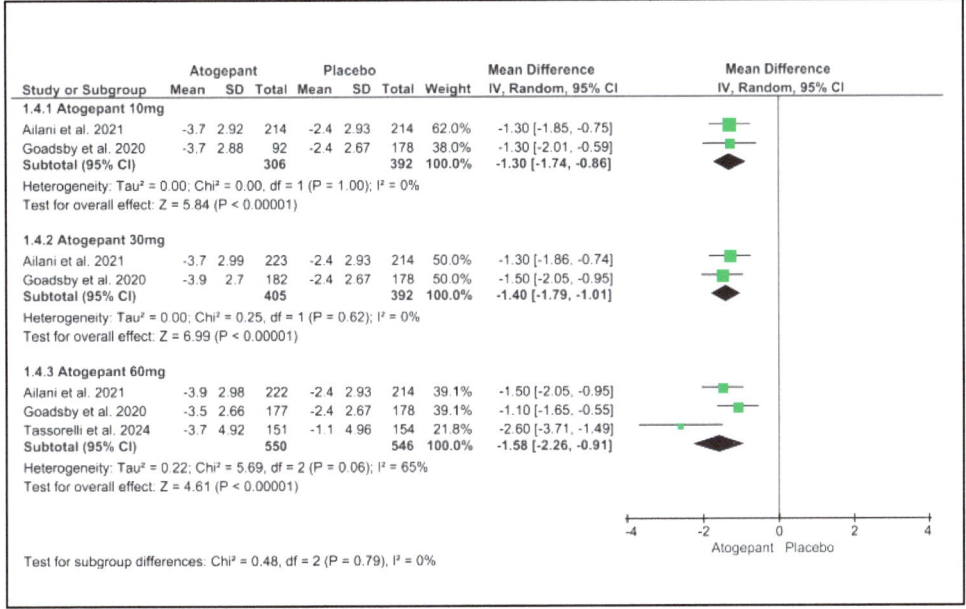

Figure 5. Acute-medications-use days change from baseline forest plot [11,26,28].

3.8. ≥Outcome of 50% Reduction in Monthly Migraine Days

A forest plot was utilized to analyze three of the selected studies, focusing on the outcome of a 50% reduction in monthly migraine days. The analysis demonstrated that, compared to a placebo, atogepant at doses of 10 mg, 30 mg, and 60 mg resulted in a reduction of more than 50% in monthly migraine days over the 12-week follow-up period. Significant heterogeneity was noted within the 30 mg and 60 mg subgroups. The relative risks (RR) for the different dosages of atogepant were as follows: 10 mg (RR = -1.66; $p = 0.003$; $I^2 = 65\%$), 30 mg (RR = 1.63; $p = 0.02$; $I^2 = 85\%$), and 60 mg (RR = 1.94; $p = 0.003$; $I^2 = 87\%$) (Figure 6).

3.9. Adverse Events

According to Goadsby et al. (2020), the incidence of treatment-emergent adverse events (TEAEs) increased with higher doses of atogepant, rising from 18% in the 10 mg once-daily subgroup to 26% in the 60 mg twice-daily subgroup, while the placebo group experienced a lower rate of 16% [26]. Nausea was identified as the most common treatment-related TEAE, occurring in 3–6% of the once-daily dose subgroups and 6–9% of the twice-daily dose subgroups, with rates ranging from 3% in the 10 mg once-daily group to 6% in the 60 mg once-daily group, compared to 3% for placebo. Notably, no evidence hepatic injury was reported [26].

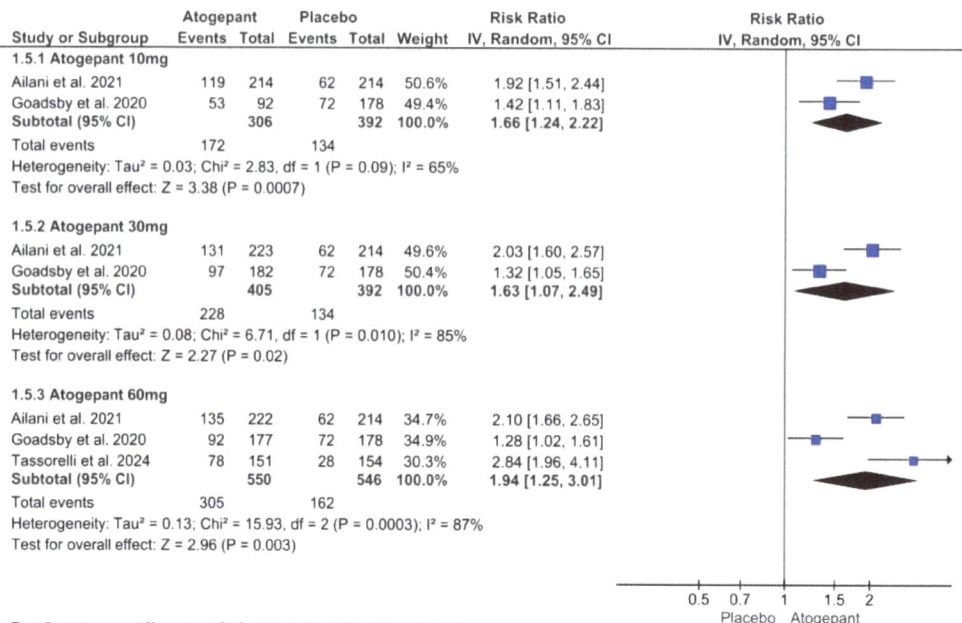

Figure 6. ≥50% reduction in monthly migraine days forest plot [11,26,28].

Schwedt et al. (2022) reported that the proportion of patients having treatment-emergent adverse events (TEAEs) was consistent across all groups, ranging from 52.2% to 53.7% in the atogepant treatment groups and 56.8% in the placebo group. Although the study was unable to specify the adverse events that caused cessation, it did indicate that 1.8–4.1% of the atogepant groups had such events, compared to 2.7% in the placebo group. A total of 486 out of 902 participants (53.9%) reported adverse events that started or got worse after the first dose of atogepant or placebo until 30 days after the final dose. The occurrence of events was comparable in both groups, and there was no dose relationship observed [25]. The most frequently reported side effects in the study by Ailani et al. (2021) were constipation (6.9% to 7.7% across atogepant dosages) and nausea (4.4% to 6.1% across atogepant doses). Ocular neuritis and asthma were among the serious adverse effects reported in the 10 mg atogepant group [11].

Lipton et al.'s 2022 trial found that the proportion of individuals experiencing TEAEs was similar across all atogepant groups (52.9% in the 10 mg group, 52.2% in the 30 mg group, and 53.7% in the 60 mg group) compared to the placebo group (56.8%) [9].

The most frequently reported TEAEs were constipation (7.7% in the 10 mg group, 7.0% in the 30 mg group, and 6.9% in the 60 mg group) and nausea (5.0% in the 10 mg group, 4.4% in the 30 mg group, and 6.1% in the 60 mg group), compared to 0.5% for constipation and 1.8% for nausea in the placebo group, respectively [9]. However, Lipton et al. (2023) did not describe any specific adverse events in their report [27].

According to a recent study by Tassorelli et al. (2024), 84 (54%) participants in the placebo group reported treatment-emergent adverse events compared to 81 (52%) in the atogepant group. Constipation was the most common TEAE with atogepant, occurring in 10% of cases versus 3% in the placebo group. Tassorelli et al. (2024) discovered that 3% of participants in the atogepant subgroup and 1% in the placebo group experienced significant adverse events, while 2% of individuals in the atogepant group and 1% in the placebo group encountered TEAEs that required treatment cessation [28] (Table 2).

Table 2. Summary of the reported treatment-related treatment emergent adverse events (TEAE).

	Study Reference	Placebo	Atogepant 10 mg Once Daily	Atogepant 30 mg Once Daily	Atogepant 60 mg Once Daily
Any treatment-related TEAE	Lipton et al.'s (2022) [9]	20/222 (9%)	51/221 (23.1%)	34/228 (14.9%)	45/231 (19.5%)
Constipation		1/222 (5%)	17/221 (7.7%)	16/228 (7%)	16/231 (6.9%)
Nausea		4/222 (1.8%)	11/221 (5%)	10/228 (4.4%)	14/231 (6.1%)
Any treatment-related TEAE	Ailani et al. (2021) [11]	20/222 (9%)	51/221 (23.1%)	34/228 (14.9%)	45/231 (19.5%)
Constipation		1/222 (0.5%)	17/221 (7.7%)	16/228 (7%)	16/231 (6.9%)
Upper respiratory tract infection		10/222 (4.5%)	9/221 (4.1%)	13/228 (5.7%)	9/231 (3.9%)
Nausea		4/222 (1.8%)	11/221 (5%)	10/228 (4.4%)	14/231 (6.1%)
Any treatment-related TEAE	Schwedt et al. (2022) [25]	56.80%	N/A	N/A	N/A
Nausea		N/A	N/A	N/A	N/A
Constipation		N/A	N/A	N/A	N/A
Fatigue		N/A	N/A	N/A	N/A
Any treatment-related TEAE	Goadsby et al. (2020) [26]	30/186 (16%)	17/93 (18%)	39/183 (21%)	42/186 (23%)
Nausea		5/186 (3%)	3/93 (3%)	10/183 (5%)	11/186 (6%)
Constipation		2/186 (1%)	1/93 (1%)	10/183 (5%)	8/186 (4%)
Fatigue		4/186 (2%)	1/93 (1%)	2/183 (1%)	4/186 (2%)
Any treatment-related TEAE	Lipton et al. (2023) [27]	N/A	N/A	N/A	N/A
Nausea		N/A	N/A	N/A	N/A
Constipation		N/A	N/A	N/A	N/A
Fatigue		N/A	N/A	N/A	N/A
Any treatment-related TEAE	Tassorelli et al. (2024) [28]	14/157 (9%)	N/A	N/A	31/156 (20%)
Constipation		3/157 (2%)	N/A	N/A	13/156 (8%)
Nausea		3/157 (2%)	N/A	N/A	8/156 (5%)
Decreased appetite		0	N/A	N/A	5/156 (3%)

Date was reported as: N (%), N/A: not applicable.

3.10. Any Adverse Events

Overall, three investigations were examined in this analysis. Although adverse events related to atogepant treatment did not increase significantly across all dosage categories, there was significant variability in the atogepant 10 mg and 30 mg subgroups. Atogepant 10 mg, 30 mg, and 60 mg had relative risks (RRs) of 1.11 ($p = 0.57$; $I^2 = 85\%$), 1.08 ($p = 0.64$; $I^2 = 85\%$), and 1.02 ($p = 0.78$; $I^2 = 29\%$). In all studies employing atogepant, the most commonly reported adverse events were nausea, constipation, and upper respiratory tract infection. Furthermore, Schwedt et al. (2022) found no difference in the occurrence of these side effects across all groups compared to the placebo [25] (Figure 7).

3.11. Serious Adverse Events

The three studies included in this forest plot on serious adverse events demonstrated that atogepant was comparable to a placebo and did not significantly increase the occurrence of such events. No discernible variation was observed across any of the groups. The results for atogepant 10 mg, 30 mg, and 60 mg were as follows: (RR = 1.00, $p = 1.00$, $I^2 = 0\%$), (RR = −0.63, $p = 0.58$, $I^2 = 0\%$), and (RR = 0.62, $p = 0.62$, $I^2 = 0\%$), respectively (Figure 8).

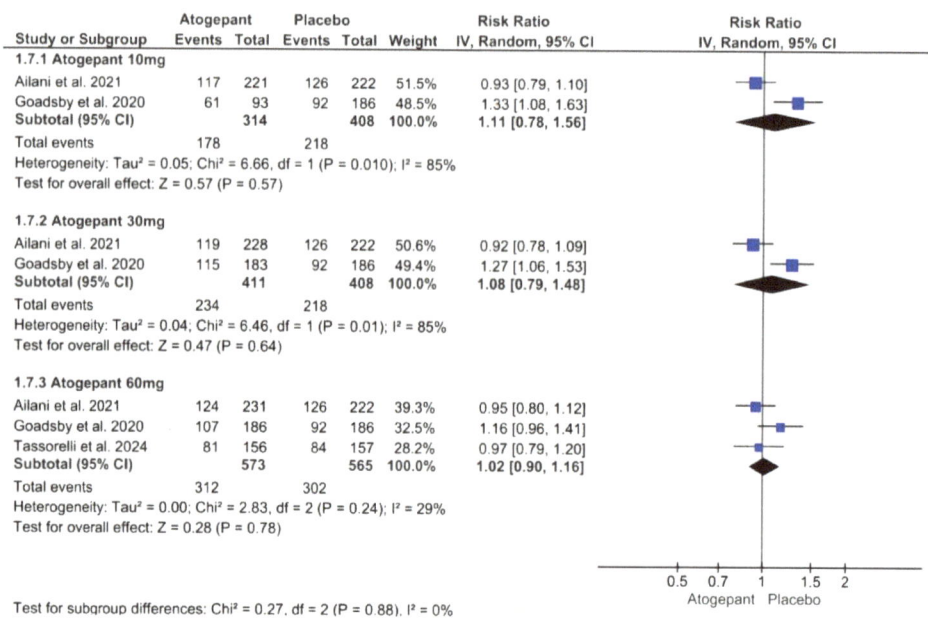

Figure 7. Any adverse events forest plot [11,26,28].

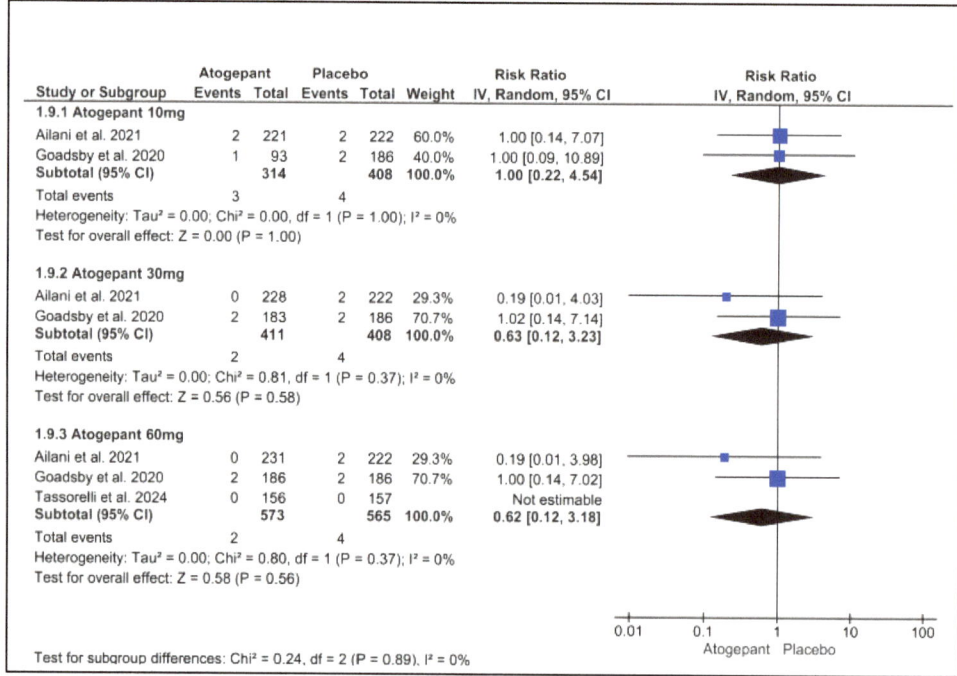

Figure 8. Serious adverse events forest plot [11,26,28].

3.12. Discontinuation Due to Adverse Events

This analysis incorporated data from five studies and determined that atogepant did not significantly increase the incidence of medication discontinuations due to adverse events in comparison to a placebo. Neither subgroup exhibited any notable heterogeneity. The three dosages of atogepant evaluated were 10 mg (RR = −1.09; p = 0.57; I^2 = 25%), 30 mg (RR = 1.01; p = 0.94; I^2 = 39%), and 60 mg (RR = 0.98; p = 0.79; I^2 = 0%). Schwedt et al. (2022) reported comparable findings, with no evidence of a dose–response relationship [25] (Figure 9).

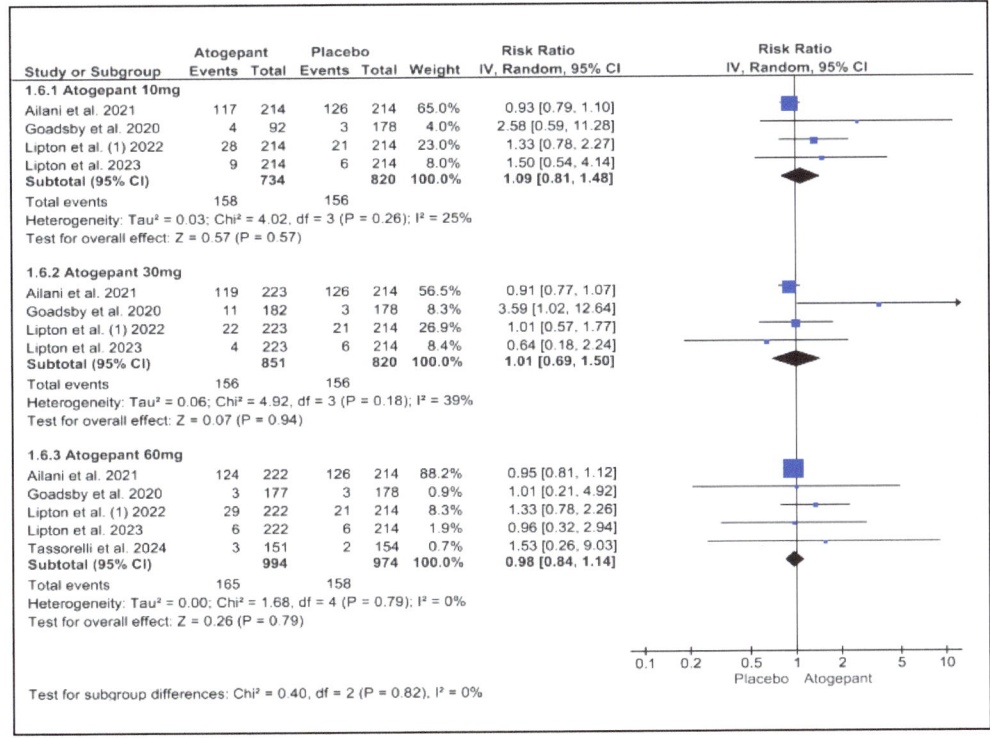

Figure 9. Discontinuation due to adverse events forest plot [9,11,26–28].

4. Discussion

In our study, we pooled data from six randomized controlled trials (RCTs) involving a total of 4569 patients to evaluate the efficacy and safety of atogepant for episodic migraine prevention. Through the analysis, different atogepant dosages (10 mg, 30 mg, and 60 mg), demonstrated that atogepant significantly reduced both mean monthly migraine days (MMDs) and mean monthly headache days (MHDs) compared to placebo over a 12-week follow-up period. The reduction was consistent across the trials, demonstrating the drug's efficacy in preventing migraines and the ability to alleviate the overall headache burden. This broader impact is particularly relevant for patients whose migraine-related disability extends beyond the headache itself, affecting overall quality of life [28].

The included trials also highlighted other key efficacy endpoints, such as the reduction in acute medication use, which is a critical factor for patients at risk of medication-overuse headaches (MOH), a common issue among migraine sufferers, which is a crucial finding, as reducing acute medication use not only alleviates symptoms but also mitigates the risk of developing MOH, which can exacerbate the condition [5]. Furthermore, the 50% responder rate analysis, which defined responders as patients achieving a ≥50% reduction in MMDs, showed significant improvements across all atogepant doses. The 10 mg dose demonstrated a relative risk of 1.66 ($p = 0.007$) compared to placebo, while the 30 mg dose showed a relative risk of 1.63 ($p = 0.02$) compared to placebo. The highest efficacy was observed with the 60 mg dose, which demonstrated a relative risk of 1.94 ($p = 0.003$) compared to placebo, indicating that higher doses yield greater benefits in terms of reduction in monthly migraine days.

According to Lipton et al. (2024), the dose–response relationship of atogepant shows that most participants who initially reported improvements continued to experience lasting benefits throughout the treatment period, particularly at higher doses. The 60 mg dose, in particular, led to better initial response rates and continued effectiveness in decreasing monthly migraine days. The data indicate that the highest dose resulted in the most participants achieving and sustaining responses at all levels of MMD reductions (50%, 75%, and 100%). These results endorse atogepant as a feasible choice for preventing episodic migraine, emphasizing the benefits of higher doses for the best treatment results [29].

When it comes to the safety profile, our review confirmed that atogepant has a favorable profile with no significant increase in adverse events compared to placebo. The most commonly reported side effects were mild, including nausea, constipation, and upper respiratory tract infections. Importantly, there was no significant dose–response relationship for adverse events, meaning that increasing the dose did not lead to a proportionate increase in adverse reactions. The absence of serious adverse events across all doses further supports atogepant's safety, making it a safer alternative to other preventive migraine therapies, such as triptans, which are often associated with cardiovascular risks [30]. This safety profile, combined with its efficacy, positions atogepant as a well-balanced option for the long-term prevention of episodic migraine.

Even though atogepant has a favorable safety profile, with no significant increase in adverse events compared to placebo, there are some reported adverse events. These findings reinforce and expand upon previous studies, establishing atogepant as an effective prophylactic treatment for episodic migraine [12,16,31,32].

The ADVANCE trial offered compelling evidence of rapid onset, with individuals having significant reductions in MMDs as early as the first week, an observation that corresponds with our findings of consistent improvements across all atogepant dosages [26]. Tassorelli et al. (2024) found that implementation of once-daily 60 mg atogepant was safe and well tolerated, and led to a significant and clinically relevant reduction in mean monthly migraine days over the course of 12 weeks when compared to placebo in patients with episodic migraine. Prior to now, two to four classes of traditional oral preventive medications had failed to achieve remission in these patients [28].

Based on estimates from the 2016 Global Burden of Disease Study, migraines rank as the second leading cause of disability-adjusted life-years (DALYs) worldwide, underscoring their substantial impact on global health [33]. Although several treatment regimens have shown efficacy in migraine prevention, there is a significant proportion of migraine patients reported to be frequent visitors of physicians' clinical practice, highlighting the urgent need to implement an efficacious and well-tolerated drug for migraine prophylaxis [5].

Atogepant, a small-molecule calcitonin gene-related peptide (CGRP) receptor antagonist, is one of the newer preventive treatments developed to manage episodic migraine. CGRP is a neuropeptide that plays a significant role in the pathophysiology of migraine, contributing to inflammation and vasodilation that can lead to headache onset [14]. By blocking the CGRP receptor, atogepant helps to prevent the onset of episodic migraine attacks. Its oral formulation allows for ease of use, particularly for patients who need daily preventive therapy. Unlike other classes of migraine treatment, such as triptans, which have vasoconstrictive properties and are associated with cardiovascular risks, atogepant does not carry such risks [5]. Furthermore, when it comes to efficacy, atogepant is found to be more effective in reducing episodic migraine attacks when compared to the other most common and non-specific migraine prophylactic drugs, such as beta-blockers and amitriptyline, making it a suitable option for a broader range of patients [34].

Studies have assessed the safety of CGRP small-molecule antagonists, called gepants, and found that they are well tolerated overall. For example, ubrogepant, one of the initial gepants authorized by the FDA, has been linked to typical side effects like nausea and drowsiness, but severe side effects are uncommon. Clinical trials show that ubrogepant has similar rates of adverse events to placebo, demonstrating its safety for treating acute migraines. Rimegepant, another type of gepant, demonstrates a comparable safety record, with the majority of negative effects being mild to moderate, such as headaches and dizziness. Both ubrogepant and rimegepant do not have significant cardiovascular risks, which makes them appropriate choices for patients with a cardiovascular history. In general, gepants offer a hopeful safety record while efficiently treating migraine episodes [30].

The American Headache Society (AHS) released a consensus statement advocating the use of CGRP-targeting medicines as a primary option for migraine prevention in addition to prior first-line therapies without requiring a prior attempt and failure of other migraine-preventive medications. The statement emphasizes the long-term tolerability and efficacy of these medications, including atogepant [35]. This conclusion was further supported by the recent 2024 National Institute for Health and Care Excellence (NICE) guidelines, which recommend atogepant as migraine preventive medication in adults who experience a minimum of four migraine days per month, but only after failing a minimum of three preventive medications [36].

Raja et al. (2024) underscore the significance of personalized treatment approaches in the management of migraines. Although all administered doses demonstrated efficacy in decreasing the number of migraine days, the analysis did not reveal a distinct dose–response relationship. Notably, higher doses, especially the 60 mg once-daily regimen, were associated with improvements in functional outcomes and a reduction in the need for acute medications, indicating a more pronounced impact on quality of life. Conversely, the efficacy of twice-daily dosing did not consistently surpass that of once-daily regimens. This suggests that lower doses may be sufficient for certain patients, while those with more severe symptoms might benefit from higher doses [37].

Previous studies, including that conducted by Tao et al. (2022) [12] and Lattanzi et al. (2022) [16] revealed that atogepant is an effective and well-tolerated episodic-migraine-preventive treatment. Furthermore, a notable heterogeneity in the ability to reduce MHDs or MMDs in the 60 mg dose group was observed, which could reflect variability in patient populations, such as demographic differences, supporting the conclusion that a personalized treatment approach may be necessary to tailor the dosage of atogepant based on individual patient factors, such as baseline migraine severity and co-morbidities. However, the findings were largely in alignment with ours; we included a greater number of RCTs and a larger sample size, which strengthened the validity of applying the results to the individual clinical practice.

In their meta-analysis, Hou et al., 2024 [31] discovered that patients who received a daily dose of atogepant 10 mg, 30 mg, or 60 mg experienced a considerably higher decrease in the mean number of migraine days from baseline than those given a placebo. Accordingly, the evaluation determined that atogepant is an effective and generally well-tolerated therapy for adult episodic migraine prophylaxis.

A recent meta-analysis conducted by Lopes et al., 2024 [32], further supported the effectiveness and tolerability of atogepant for migraine prevention, including episodic or chronic migraine, when compared to placebo. They noticed that in terms of the monthly reduction of migraine or headache days, the overall impact estimate of atogepant was much greater than that of placebo.

Although our findings back up these recent meta-analyses' findings [31,32], our meta-analysis offers a more focused assessment by exclusively including episodic migraine patients. This specificity enhances the accuracy of the findings for this patient population. The inclusion of both episodic and chronic migraine populations may have diluted the efficacy results for episodic migraine. By focusing solely on episodic migraine, we provide more reliable and precise insights into the efficacy of atogepant for this group, considering the different pathophysiological features of chronic when compared to episodic migraines.

Strengths and Limitations

Compared to the current literature, our study provides a comprehensive and focused assessment by including only studies that specifically evaluate the safety and efficacy of atogepant in episodic migraine patients. However, several limitations should be noted: Firstly, the meta-analysis incorporated a relatively small number of randomized controlled trials (RCTs) with a short follow-up period of 12 weeks. These factors may constrain the applicability of the results to wider contexts. This brief period may not be sufficient for assessing atogepant's long-term safety and efficacy, especially for chronic conditions such as migraine that require ongoing treatment. One important limitation is the absence of extended safety evaluations, making it harder to predict potential late-onset side effects and the lasting effectiveness of medical results.

Furthermore, the results may not be as broadly applicable, as they may be due to different demographic considerations, since all the research efforts were carried out in Western nations. Finally, the lack of sufficient reported outcomes made it difficult to perform a meta-analysis of adverse events (AEs).

5. Conclusions

In patients with episodic migraine, atogepant has shown notable effectiveness in lowering MMDs, MHDs, and acute drug use while raising the 50% responder rate. The need for individualized treatment plans is highlighted by the observed variability in the higher-dose groups. To verify atogepant's long-term effectiveness and safety, especially in larger patient groups, and to evaluate its possible function in conjunction with other treatments for the best migraine care, more extensive clinical trials are required. Future research should consider geographical and demographic differences across populations to help shape a new era of personalized treatment approaches.

Author Contributions: Conceptualization: A.S.A.; Methodology: A.S.A., T.M.A., and R.A.A.; Software: A.S.A., T.M.A., R.A.A., N.M.A., and M.M.A.; Validation: A.S.A., T.M.A., and R.A.A.; Formal Analysis: A.S.A.; Investigation: A.S.A., T.M.A., R.A.A., N.M.A., and M.M.A.; Resources: A.S.A., N.M.A., and M.M.A.; Data Curation: A.S.A., T.M.A., R.A.A., N.M.A., and M.M.A.; Writing—Original Draft Preparation: A.S.A., T.M.A., R.A.A., N.M.A., and M.M.A.; Writing—Review & Editing: A.S.A., T.M.A., R.A.A., N.M.A., and M.M.A.; Visualization: A.S.A.; Supervision: M.M.A.; Project Administration: A.S.A., T.M.A., R.A.A., N.M.A., and M.M.A.; Funding Acquisition: M.M.A. All authors have read and agreed to the published version of the manuscript.

Funding: This research received no external funding.

Institutional Review Board Statement: Ethical review and approval were waived for this study due to study design.

Informed Consent Statement: Not applicable.

Data Availability Statement: The original contributions presented in the study are included in the article. Further inquiries can be directed to the corresponding author.

Conflicts of Interest: The authors declare no conflicts of interest.

References

1. Lipton, R.B.; Bigal, M.E.; Diamond, M.; Freitag, F.; Reed, M.L.; Stewart, W.F. Migraine prevalence, disease burden, and the need for preventive therapy. *Neurology* **2007**, *68*, 343–349. Available online: https://www.neurology.org/doi/10.1212/01.wnl.0000252808.97649.21?url_ver=Z39.88-2003&rfr_id=ori:rid:crossref.org&rfr_dat=cr_pub%20%200pubmed (accessed on 30 June 2024). [CrossRef] [PubMed]
2. Steiner, T.J.; Stovner, L.J.; Birbeck, G.L. Migraine: The seventh disabler. *J. Headache Pain* **2013**, *14*, 1–3. Available online: https://www.ncbi.nlm.nih.gov/pmc/articles/PMC3606966/pdf/1129-2377-14-1.pdf (accessed on 30 June 2024). [CrossRef] [PubMed]

3. Steiner, T.J.; Stovner, L.J.; Jensen, R.; Uluduz, D.; Katsarava, Z. Migraine remains second among the world's causes of disability, and first among young women: Findings from GBD2019. *Headache Pain* **2020**, *21*, 137–141. Available online: https://www.ncbi.nlm.nih.gov/pmc/articles/PMC7708887/pdf/10194_2020_Article_1208.pdf (accessed on 30 June 2024). [CrossRef]
4. Stewart, W.F.; Ricci, J.A.; Chee, E.; Morganstein, D.; Lipton, R. Lost Productive Time and Cost Due to Common Pain Conditions in the US Workforce. *JAMA* **2003**, *290*, 2443–2454. Available online: https://jamanetwork.com/journals/jama/fullarticle/197628#google_vignette (accessed on 30 June 2024). [CrossRef]
5. Ashina, M.; Katsarava, Z.; Do, T.P.; Buse, D.C.; Pozo-Rosich, P.; Özge, A.; Krymchantowski, A.V.; Lebedeva, E.R.; Ravishankar, K.; Yu, S.; et al. Migraine: Epidemiology and systems of care. *Lancet* **2021**, *397*, 1485–1495. Available online: https://www.thelancet.com/journals/lancet/article/PIIS0140-6736(20)32160-7/abstract (accessed on 30 June 2024). [CrossRef]
6. Leonardi, M.; Raggi, A. Burden of migraine: International perspectives. *Neurol. Sci.* **2013**, *34* (Suppl. S1), S117–S118. Available online: https://link.springer.com/article/10.1007/s10072-013-1387-8 (accessed on 30 June 2024). [CrossRef]
7. Olesen, J.; Headache Classification Committee of the International Headache Society (IHS). The International Classification of Headache Disorders, 3rd edition. *Cephalalgia* **2018**, *1*, 1–211. Available online: https://www.ichd-3.org/wp-content/uploads/2018/01/The-International-Classification-of-Headache-Disorders-3rd-Edition-2018.pdf (accessed on 30 June 2024).
8. Buse, D.C.; Manack, A.N.; Fanning, K.M.; Serrano, D.; Reed, M.L.; Turkel, C.C.; Lipton, R.B. Chronic migraine prevalence, disability, and sociodemographic factors: Results from the American migraine prevalence and prevention study. *Headache* **2012**, *52*, 1456–1470. Available online: https://headachejournal.onlinelibrary.wiley.com/doi/epdf/10.1111/j.1526-4610.2012.02223.x (accessed on 30 June 2024). [CrossRef]
9. Lipton, R.B.; Pozo-Rosich, P.; Blumenfeld, A.M.; Dodick, D.W.; McAllister, P.; Li, Y.; Lu, K.; Dabruzzo, B.; Miceli, R.; Severt, L.; et al. Rates of Response to Atogepant for Migraine Prophylaxis among Adults: A Secondary Analysis of a Randomized Clinical Trial. *JAMA Netw. Open* **2022**, *5*, E2215499. Available online: https://www.ncbi.nlm.nih.gov/pmc/articles/PMC9178435/#:~:text=In%20a%20secondary%20analysis%20of%20a%20phase%203,,mean%20monthly%20migraine-days%20during%202012%20weeks%20of%20treatment (accessed on 30 June 2024). [CrossRef]
10. Katsarava, Z.; Buse, D.C.; Manack, A.N.; Lipton, R.B. Defining the differences between episodic migraine and chronic migraine. *Curr. Pain Headache Rep.* **2012**, *16*, 86–92. Available online: https://www.ncbi.nlm.nih.gov/pmc/articles/PMC3258393/pdf/11916_2011_Article_233.pdf (accessed on 30 June 2024). [CrossRef]
11. Ailani, J.; Lipton, R.B.; Goadsby, P.J.; Guo, H.; Miceli, R.; Severt, L.; Finnegan, M.; Trugman, J.M.; ADVANCE Study Group. Atogepant for the Preventive Treatment of Migraine. *N. Engl. J. Med.* **2021**, *385*, 695–706. Available online: https://www.nejm.org/doi/pdf/10.1056/NEJMoa2035908 (accessed on 30 June 2024). [CrossRef] [PubMed]
12. Tao, X.; Yan, Z.; Meng, J.; Wang, W.; Dai, Q.; Zhou, Q.; Wang, Z.; Wang, Z. The efficacy and safety of atogepant for the prophylactic treatment of migraine: Evidence from randomized controlled trials. *J. Headache Pain* **2022**, *23*, 19–31. Available online: https://www.ncbi.nlm.nih.gov/pmc/articles/PMC8903713/pdf/10194_2022_Article_1391.pdf (accessed on 30 June 2024). [CrossRef] [PubMed]
13. Sacco, S.; Lampl, C.; Maassen van den Brink, A.; Caponnetto, V.; Braschinsky, M.; Ducros, A.; Little, P.; Pozo-Rosich, P.; Reuter, U.; Ruiz de la Torre, E.; et al. Burden and Attitude to Resistant and Refractory (BARR) Study Group; Burden and attitude to resistant and refractory migraine: A survey from the European Headache Federation with the endorsement of the European Migraine & Headache Alliance. *J. Headache Pain* **2021**, *22*, 39–49. Available online: https://www.ncbi.nlm.nih.gov/pmc/articles/PMC8130435/pdf/10194_2021_Article_1252.pdf (accessed on 30 June 2024). [PubMed]
14. Goadsby, P.J.; Holland, P.R.; Martins-Oliveira, M.; Hoffmann, J.; Schankin, C.; Akerman, S. Pathophysiology of Migraine: A Disorder of Sensory Processing. *Physiol. Rev.* **2017**, *97*, 553–622. Available online: https://www.ncbi.nlm.nih.gov/pmc/articles/PMC5539409/ (accessed on 30 June 2024). [CrossRef]
15. Dodick, D.W. Migraine. *Lancet* **2018**, *391*, 1315–1330. [CrossRef]
16. Lattanzi, S.; Trinka, E.; Altamura, C.; Del Giovane, C.; Silvestrini, M.; Brigo, F.; Vernieri, F. Atogepant for the Prevention of Episodic Migraine in Adults: A Systematic Review and Meta-Analysis of Efficacy and Safety. *Neurol. Ther.* **2022**, *11*, 1235–1252. Available online: https://link.springer.com/content/pdf/10.1007/s40120-022-00370-8.pdf (accessed on 30 June 2024). [CrossRef]
17. Tepper, D. Gepants. Headache: The Journal of Head and Face Pain© 2020 American Headache Society Published by Wiley Periodicals, Inc. 1037–1039. Available online: https://headachejournal.onlinelibrary.wiley.com/doi/epdf/10.1111/head.13791 (accessed on 30 June 2024).
18. Tassorelli, C.; Onishchenko, K.; Halker Singh, R.B.; Duan, M.; Dupont-Benjamin, L.; Hemstock, M.; Voller, C.; McAllister, P.; Nahas, S.J.; Gandhi, P.; et al. Comparative efficacy, quality of life, safety, and tolerability of atogepant and rimegepant in migraine prevention: A matching-adjusted indirect comparison analysis. *Cephalalgia* **2024**, *44*, 3331024241235156. [CrossRef]
19. Switzer, M.P.; Robinson, J.E.; Joyner, K.R.; Morgan, K.W. Atogepant for the prevention of episodic migraine in adults. *SAGE Open Med.* **2022**, *10*, 20503121221128688. [CrossRef]
20. Schiffman, E.; Ohrbach, R.; Truelove, E.; Anderson, G.; Goulet, J.-P.; List, T.; Svensson, P.; Gonzalez, Y.; Lobbezoo, F.; Michelotti, A.; et al. The International Classification of Headache Disorders, 3rd edition (beta version). *Cephalalgia* **2013**, *33*, 629–808. Available online: https://www.zora.uzh.ch/id/eprint/89115/ (accessed on 30 June 2024).
21. Seo, H.J.; Kim, S.Y.; Lee, Y.J.; Park, J.E. RoBANS 2: A Revised Risk of Bias Assessment Tool for Nonrandomized Studies of Interventions. *Korean J. Fam. Med.* **2023**, *44*, 249–260. Available online: https://www.ncbi.nlm.nih.gov/pmc/articles/PMC10522469/pdf/kjfm-23-0034.pdf (accessed on 30 June 2024). [CrossRef]

22. Sterne, J.A.C.; Savović, J.; Page, M.J.; Elbers, R.G.; Blencowe, N.S.; Boutron, I.; Cates, C.J.; Cheng, H.Y.; Corbett, M.S.; Eldridge, S.M.; et al. RoB 2: A revised tool for assessing risk of bias in randomised trials. *BMJ* **2019**, *366*, l4898. Available online: https://www.bmj.com/content/bmj/366/bmj.l4898.full.pdf (accessed on 30 June 2024). [CrossRef] [PubMed]
23. Higgins, J.P.T.; Thompson, S.G. Quantifying heterogeneity in a meta-analysis. *Stat. Med.* **2002**, *21*, 1539–1558. Available online: https://pubmed.ncbi.nlm.nih.gov/12111919/ (accessed on 30 June 2024). [CrossRef] [PubMed]
24. Book Series, C.; Higgins, J.P.; Green, S. *Cochrane Handbook for Systematic Reviews of Interventions*; The Cochrane Collaboration®: London, UK, 2008.
25. Schwedt, T.J.; Lipton, R.B.; Ailani, J.; Silberstein, S.D.; Tassorelli, C.; Guo, H.; Lu, K.; Dabruzzo, B.; Miceli, R.; Severt, L.; et al. Time course of efficacy of atogepant for the preventive treatment of migraine: Results from the randomized, double-blind ADVANCE trial. *Cephalalgia* **2022**, *42*, 3–11. Available online: https://www.ncbi.nlm.nih.gov/pmc/articles/PMC8739573/pdf/10.1177_03331024211042385.pdf (accessed on 30 June 2024). [CrossRef] [PubMed]
26. Goadsby, P.J.; Dodick, D.W.; Ailani, J.; Trugman, J.M.; Finnegan, M.; Lu, K.; Szegedi, A. Safety, tolerability, and efficacy of orally administered atogepant for the prevention of episodic migraine in adults: A double-blind, randomised phase 2b/3 trial. *Lancet Neurol.* **2020**, *19*, 727–737. Available online: https://www.thelancet.com/journals/laneur/article/PIIS1474-4422(20)30234-9/abstract (accessed on 30 June 2024). [CrossRef]
27. Lipton, R.B.; Pozo-Rosich, P.; Blumenfeld, A.M.; Li, Y.; Severt, L.; Stokes, J.T.; Creutz, L.; Gandhi, P.; Dodick, D. Effect of Atogepant for Preventive Migraine Treatment on Patient-Reported Outcomes in the Randomized, Double-blind, Phase 3 ADVANCE Trial. *Neurology* **2023**, *100*, E764–E777. Available online: https://www.ncbi.nlm.nih.gov/pmc/articles/PMC9984220/pdf/WNL-2022-201407.pdf (accessed on 30 June 2024). [CrossRef]
28. Tassorelli, C.; Nagy, K.; Pozo-Rosich, P.; Lanteri-Minet, M.; Sacco, S.; Nežádal, T.; Guo, H.; De Abreu Ferreira, R.; Forero, G.; Trugman, J.M. Safety and efficacy of atogepant for the preventive treatment of episodic migraine in adults for whom conventional oral preventive treatments have failed (ELEVATE): A randomised, placebo-controlled, phase 3b trial. *Lancet Neurol.* **2024**, *23*, 382–392. Available online: https://www.thelancet.com/journals/laneur/article/PIIS1474-4422(24)00025-5/abstract (accessed on 30 June 2024). [CrossRef]
29. Lipton, R.B.; Nahas, S.J.; Pozo-Rosich, P.; Bilchik, T.; McAllister, P.; Finnegan, M.; Liu, Y.; Chalermpalanupap, N.; Dabruzzo, B.; Dodick, D.W. Sustained response to atogepant in episodic migraine: Post hoc analyses of a 12-week randomized trial and a 52-week long-term safety trial. *J. Headache Pain* **2024**, *25*, 83–94. [CrossRef]
30. Cohen, F.; Yuan, H.; Silberstein, S.D. Calcitonin Gene-Related Peptide (CGRP)-Targeted Monoclonal Antibodies and Antagonists in Migraine: Current Evidence and Rationale. *BioDrugs* **2022**, *36*, 341–358. [CrossRef]
31. Hou, M.; Luo, X.; He, S.; Yang, X.; Zhang, Q.; Jin, M.; Zhang, P.; Li, Y.; Bi, X.; Li, J.; et al. Efficacy and safety of atogepant, a small molecule CGRP receptor antagonist, for the preventive treatment of migraine: A systematic review and meta-analysis. *J. Headache Pain* **2024**, *25*, 116–132. Available online: https://www.ncbi.nlm.nih.gov/pmc/articles/PMC11264921/pdf/10194_2024_Article_1822.pdf (accessed on 30 June 2024). [CrossRef]
32. Lopes, L.M.; de Almeida, A.M.; Pasqualotto, E.; Sudo, R.Y.; Leite, M.G.; Souza, M.E.C.; de Moraes, F.C.A.; Siebel, V.M.; Figueiredo, N. Efficacy and Safety of Atogepant for Preventing Chronic and Episodic Migraines: A Systematic Review and Meta-Analysis of Randomized Controlled Trials. *Curr. Treat. Options Neurol.* **2024**, *26*, 411–419. Available online: https://link.springer.com/article/10.1007/s11940-024-00803-9 (accessed on 30 June 2024). [CrossRef]
33. Feigin, V.L.; Nichols, E.; Alam, T.; Bannick, M.S.; Beghi, E.; Blake, N.; Culpepper, W.J.; Dorsey, E.R.; Elbaz, A.; Ellenbogen, R.G.; et al. Global, regional, and national burden of neurological disorders, 1990–2016: A systematic analysis for the Global Burden of Disease Study 2016. *Lancet Neurol.* **2019**, *18*, 459–480. Available online: https://research.wur.nl/en/publications/global-regional-and-national-burden-of-neurological-disorders-199 (accessed on 30 June 2024). [CrossRef] [PubMed]
34. Lampl, C.; Maassen Van Den Brink, A.; Deligianni, C.I.; Gil-Gouveia, R.; Jassal, T.; Sanchez-del-Rio, M.; Reuter, U.; Uluduz, D.; Versijpt, J.; Zeraatkar, D.; et al. The comparative effectiveness of migraine preventive drugs: A systematic review and network meta-analysis. *J. Headache Pain* **2023**, *24*, 56–70. Available online: https://www.ncbi.nlm.nih.gov/pmc/articles/PMC10197489/pdf/10194_2023_Article_1594.pdf (accessed on 30 June 2024). [CrossRef] [PubMed]
35. Charles, A.C.; Digre, K.B.; Goadsby, P.J.; Robbins, M.S.; Hershey, A. American Headache Society.; Calcitonin gene-related peptide-targeting therapies are a first-line option for the prevention of migraine: An American Headache Society position statement update. *Headache* **2024**, *64*, 333–341. Available online: https://headachejournal.onlinelibrary.wiley.com/doi/epdf/10.1111/head.14692 (accessed on 30 June 2024). [CrossRef] [PubMed]
36. National Institute for Health and Care Excellence (NICE). Atogepant for Preventing Migraine Technology Appraisal Guidance. 2024. Available online: https://www.nice.org.uk/guidance/ta973/resources/atogepant-for-preventing-migraine-pdf-82615848254917 (accessed on 30 June 2024).
37. Raja, A.; Asim, R.; Shuja, M.H.; Raja, S.; Saleh Muhammad, T.; Bajaj, S.; Ansari, A.H.; Ali, H.; Magsi, I.A.; Faridi, M.H.; et al. Atogepant for Migraine Prevention: A Meta-Analysis of Safety and Efficacy in Adults. *Front. Neurol.* **2024**, *15*, 1468961. [CrossRef]

Disclaimer/Publisher's Note: The statements, opinions and data contained in all publications are solely those of the individual author(s) and contributor(s) and not of MDPI and/or the editor(s). MDPI and/or the editor(s) disclaim responsibility for any injury to people or property resulting from any ideas, methods, instructions or products referred to in the content.

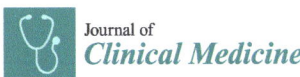

Review

Telecoaching and Migraine: Digital Approach to Physical Activity in Migraine Management. A Scoping Review

Ignazio Leale [1,2,*], Vincenzo Di Stefano [3], Angelo Torrente [3], Paolo Alonge [3], Roberto Monastero [3], Michele Roccella [2], Filippo Brighina [3], Valerio Giustino [1,2] and Giuseppe Battaglia [1,2]

[1] Sport and Exercise Research Unit, Department of Psychology, Educational Sciences and Human Movement, University of Palermo, 90144 Palermo, Italy; valerio.giustino@unipa.it (V.G.); giuseppe.battaglia@unipa.it (G.B.)
[2] Department of Psychology, Educational Science and Human Movement, University of Palermo, 90129 Palermo, Italy; michele.roccella@unipa.it
[3] Department of Biomedicine, Neuroscience, and Advanced Diagnostics (BiND), University of Palermo, 90129 Palermo, Italy; vincenzo.distefano07@unipa.it (V.D.S.); angelo.torrente@unipa.it (A.T.); paolo.alonge01@unipa.it (P.A.); roberto.monastero@unipa.it (R.M.); filippo.brighina@unipa.it (F.B.)
* Correspondence: ignazio.leale@unipa.it

Abstract: Migraine is a common neurological disorder, affecting approximately 15% of the European population and is among the main causes of years lived with disability. In the context of increasing digitalisation, telecoaching (TC) is a new training modality that involves the use of digital tools to access and manage training services remotely. Given the well-documented benefits of physical activity in migraine management and the rapid expansion of digital health services following the COVID-19 pandemic, this scoping review aims to evaluate the use and feasibility of TC-based training programs in individuals with migraine. A systematic search was conducted on multiple databases (PubMed, Web of Science, and Scopus) identifying 1507 studies, of which only 3 met the inclusion criteria. These studies collectively involved 181 participants with migraine and assessed various training programs, including aerobic training, resistance training, and physical therapy. Most training programs showed statistically significant improvements in several variables, including severity, duration, and frequency of migraine attacks. However, based on our study, there is limited evidence to suggest that TC training is beneficial for migraine patients. These findings underscore the need for further investigation, with more rigorous methodologies, higher-quality trials, and larger sample sizes to better establish the efficacy of TC training as a preventive and therapeutic approach for migraine.

Keywords: telecoaching; migraine; adapted physical activity; exercise; digital tools; COVID-19; lifestyle changes

1. Introduction

1.1. Incidence and Impact of Migraine

Migraine is a highly common neurological disorder that affects approximately 15% of the European population [1], resulting in the second most severe disorder in terms of years lived with disability [2], and is the main cause of disability in the 15–49 age group [2]. It is a cyclic disorder characterised by recurrent attacks of moderate-to-severe headaches that may be pulsating in quality and unilateral, accompanied by nausea and intolerance to light or noise [3]. Moreover, one of the characteristics is that the pain usually worsens with physical exercise [3]. Some patients also experience transient focal neurological symptoms (usually lasting up to one hour each) before or during an attack, called aura, which configure the migraine with aura subtype [3].

Migraine creates a debilitating condition that causes work absenteeism or presenteeism (i.e., working with limited efficiency) and reduced participation in social activities [4]. Some consequences are high economic losses [5] and an increased risk of side effects due to overuse or misuse of medications [6].

1.2. Pathogenesis and Management of Migraine

In recent decades, much progress has been made in understanding the physiopathology, genetics, and neurophysiology of migraine. There is strong evidence that migraine may depend on alterations in cortical excitability (i.e., increased), which may lead to maladaptive patterns of brain plasticity, especially when the frequency of headache attacks increases (i.e., transformation from episodic to chronic migraine) [7–9].

The progress allowed the creation of new opportunities for the diagnosis and management of this disorder, even in rare familial forms [10,11]. There are two different approaches, which include the use of acute medication to stop a migraine attack, or preventive medication to reduce the frequency, duration, and severity of the pain episodes. The guidelines recommend the use of preventatives in case of debilitating headaches occurring for 2 or more days per month [12]. However, traditional oral prophylaxes may not be well tolerated or accepted by patients due to the possible side effects [13,14].

1.3. Non-Pharmacological Treatment of Migraine

For the above-mentioned reasons, non-pharmacological treatments, such as self-management strategies, manual therapy, physical activity, or physical exercise progressively gained interest as valid alternatives to conventional therapies [15–17]. Sport has a controversial role in migraine [18,19]. Although sport has been associated with a worsening of migraine attacks [20,21], there is evidence that regular physical activity or physical exercise could play a primary role in preventing them [22,23]. This phenomenon could be related to the intensity of exercise. High-intensity exercise (mainly present in sport) is a migraine trigger [20,21], while regular and moderate-intensity exercise (mainly present in physical activity) plays a role in attacks prevention [19,23]. Busch and colleagues [23], in their review, showed that regular, planned, and structured physical activity was associated with several benefits in this target population. The beneficial effects of exercise on migraine may be related to better pain modulation. Indeed, several studies demonstrate the analgesic effect of aerobic exercise [24,25]. Despite these findings, it has been shown that patients with migraine are more sedentary than healthy subjects [26]; a sedentary lifestyle that has further increased due to the recent COVID-19 pandemic, in several neurological disorders [27,28]. On the other side, the recent COVID-19 pandemic raised the need and gave impulse for the development of telemedicine.

1.4. Aerobic and Resistance Training: Evidence-Based Benefits

Recent literature demonstrated that exercise plays a significant role in the management of migraine. Specifically, aerobic activity has been shown to be particularly effective in reducing both the frequency and intensity of headache episodes, as well as enhancing the overall well-being of patients [29,30]. Indeed, as shown by the current literature, aerobic activity improves not only the specific parameters of migraine (frequency, intensity, and duration), but also the cardiovascular function, the affective discomfort [30], and the quality of life (QoL) of these patients [29]. A recent systematic review highlighted that moderate aerobic training is the most effective approach for reducing migraine-related disability [31]. Furthermore, the findings suggest that combining pharmacological treatment with aerobic training is more effective than drug treatment alone in decreasing both the frequency and intensity of migraine attacks [31].

Resistance training has been shown to positively contribute to migraine management by enhancing overall muscle strength and physical resilience, as well as reducing the frequency of headache attacks [32]. Muscle strengthening and reconditioning, particularly focused on the neck, shoulder, and upper limb muscles, could be the mechanisms responsible for the therapeutic effects of resistance training [32]. Furthermore, resistance training facilitates the increase and preservation of lean muscle mass, which can help reduce sarcopenia [33]. Research indicates that an increase in lean muscle mass is associated with a reduction in the frequency of migraine episodes [34]. These findings highlight the importance of incorporating resistance training into a comprehensive approach to migraine management.

1.5. Telecoaching: New Training Approach

A recent study showed the important association between migraine and some neurodegenerative disorders. For example, patients with migraine are more likely to develop Parkinson's disease (PD) than subjects without migraine [35]. Kim and colleagues also found a relevant association between migraine and Alzheimer's disease [36]. The authors demonstrated that individuals with a history of migraine had a higher prevalence of Alzheimer's disease. The association was even stronger in young and obese subjects with migraine [36]. These findings suggest that migraine may be a risk factor for some neurodegenerative diseases, so proper migraine management (as well as an active lifestyle) might help reduce this risk. For these reasons, there is a need to develop new intervention strategies to contrast migraine and increase physical activity levels. This approach could also induce changes in brain plasticity that could have a beneficial effect on headache frequency.

A new training modality could be represented by telecoaching (TC). Unlike traditional training, where exercises are performed in specific facilities and coach–athlete communication occurs in person, TC utilises technological and digital tools, such as computers and mobile devices, to deliver and manage training services remotely. This new approach of distance communication offers greater flexibility and facilitates access to the training. Technological tools allow the trainer to send training materials and monitor adherence to the program, while allowing patients to train independently, overcoming obstacles such as time, distances, and transport [37]. This new approach could serve as a primary strategy to increase adherence and engagement of individuals, reducing sedentary lifestyles. The effectiveness of TC in other populations and diseases has already been demonstrated, including its efficacy in the elderly population [38,39], in respiratory diseases [40,41], in patients with metabolic or cardiac diseases [42,43], as well as in patients with other neurological diseases such as Charcot–Marie–Tooth [44,45]. Therefore, TC could be one of the main tools to be used to increase physical activity levels in migraine patients, reducing their sedentary lifestyle and promoting improved QoL, autonomy, and self-esteem [46]. However, potential issues related to internet connection, as well as video and audio quality, should be considered to ensure the effectiveness of this modality [47]. TC aligns well with telemedicine and eHealth, which, despite its various approaches and challenges primarily related to the complexities of app development [48], has been extensively utilised and studied [47], as well as with the use of wearable devices for the benefit of human health [49]. While some patients express a preference for a hybrid care model [48], telemedicine consultations demonstrated a quality of care comparable to that of traditional headache outpatient consultations, offering a more cost-effective solution for patients [47], with also a positive endorsement from neurologists [50]. However, the use of telemedicine is significantly influenced by geographic location [51]. Countries such as the United States, China, and Norway, which benefit from advanced technology, make extensive use of telemedicine [52,53]. In contrast, countries such as Lithuania have not adopted this tool to the same extent. A recent study indicated that only 17% of migraine patients in Lithuania received remote consultations, compared to 57.5% of patients in the United States [51,52]. Positive experiences with telemedicine may encourage wider adoption of this approach.

1.6. Aim of the Study

Considering these premises, this scoping review aims to identify the available evidence on the use and feasibility of TC training programs in migraine patients.

2. Materials and Methods

This scoping review was developed according to the PRISMA guidelines for systematic reviews and meta-analysis [54]. The protocol was not recorded in a specific database but was developed before the study.

2.1. Eligibility Criteria

Inclusion criteria were: (a) original research with full text written in English; (b) all study designs different than reviews, meta-analyses, letters to editors, and theses; (c) studies with training programs performed in TC for migraine patients; (d) studies published over the last decade, concluding in September 2024. No gender difference between males and females was used as an exclusion criterion. The population, intervention, comparison, outcome, and study design (PICOS) framework was used as shown in Table 1.

Table 1. The PICOS framework.

PICOS Components	Details
Population	Individuals with migraine.
Intervention	Telecoaching training program (aerobic training, resistance training, stretching, and physical therapy).
Comparison	The post-exercise migraine endpoints were compared to pre-exercise migraine endpoints within each study.
Outcome	Migraine endpoints (migraine days, attack frequency, pain intensity, and duration of migraine attacks).
Study design	Original articles.

2.2. Data Collection

Major databases, including PubMed (NLM), Web of Science (TS), and Scopus, were used to find useful articles for this study. Keywords included: exercise, physical activity, telecoaching, migraine, and headache. The different terms have been divided into 3 groups. In Group A, the terms "migraine" and "headache" were entered; in Group B, the terms "exercise" and "physical activity"; and in Group C, the term "telecoaching" was entered. The Boolean operators 'AND' and 'OR' were used to analyse the three categories. Matching examples were "migraine" AND "physical activity" AND "telecoaching". All items found were transferred to Endnote software for the analyses (Version X20 for Windows 11, Thomson Reuters, New York, NY, USA).

2.2.1. Study Selection

Database analysis, identification, and elimination of duplicates were carried out by a single researcher. Subsequently, two authors independently analysed the studies (I.L.; V.D.S.). In detail, in the initial phase, the title and abstract of each study was examined; in the final phase, the researchers double-checked the entire text to confirm that the selected studies met the inclusion and exclusion criteria. In case of disagreements between the two raters on the inclusion or exclusion of a study, a third researcher was consulted (G.B). A Microsoft Excel spreadsheet (Microsoft Corp, Redmond, WA, USA) was used to report the study information including year of publication, age of sample, gender, aim of the study, results, and TC training protocol. The PRISMA flow diagram (Figure 1) illustrates the process by which the articles were selected.

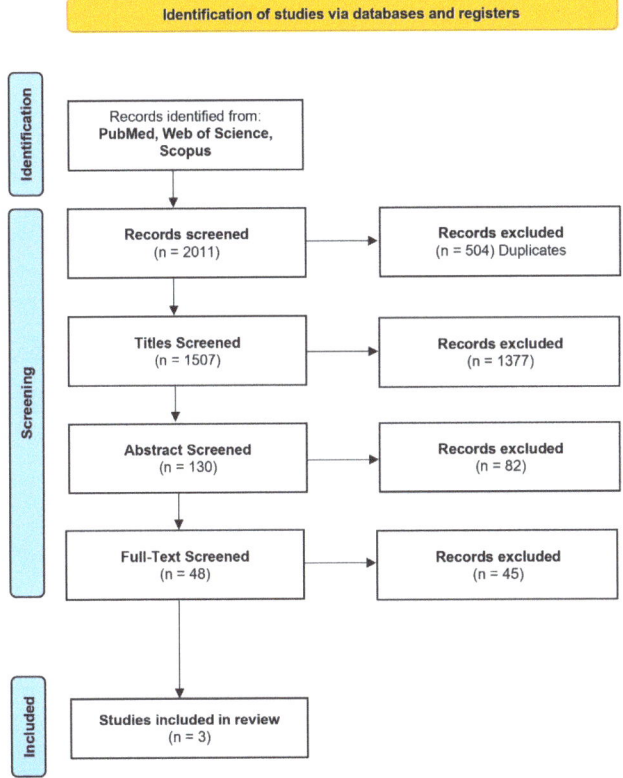

Figure 1. The flow diagram representing the selection process of records.

2.2.2. Quality and Risk of Bias Assessment

Two authors (I.L.; V.D.S.) evaluated the quality and BIAS of all the studies included, using a modified version of the "Downs and Black Checklist" [55]. In the modified version of the Downs and Black checklist, the score of item 27 (concerning the power of the study) was changed from 0–5 to 0–1, so that a study would receive a score of 0 in case the statistical power was below 80%, and a score of 1 if the statistical power was above 80% [56]. Taking this into account, the final checklist score changed from 32 to 28. The quality of the studies was divided into four levels: excellent (26–28), good (20–25), fair (15–19), and poor (<14) [57,58]. Another researcher (G.B.) compared the authors' results for each study and discrepancies were resolved through a consensus meeting.

3. Results

3.1. Study Identification

A total of 2011 studies were identified through electronic databases. In total, 504 studies were eliminated because they were duplicates; 1507 titles and 130 abstracts were analysed. The full text of 48 studies was analysed; of these, only 3 studies agreed with the inclusion and exclusion criteria. Specifically, the three included studies analysed the efficacy of a TC aerobic training program [59], a TC resistance training program [60], and a TC physical therapy [61]. A total of 181 participants with migraine were included in this review. All included studies presented data on both males and females, but female sex was prevalent (n = 139, 76.7%). More detailed information about the study selection process and the characteristics of the included studies can be found in Figure 1 and Table 2.

Table 2. The aim of the studies and relative characteristics of the samples.

First Author, Year	Participants [F%], Age ± SD	Aim	Telecoaching Strategies	Downs and Black Score
Santiago, 2014 [59]	60 [88%], 31 ± 9	To compare the preventive treatment benefits of amitriptyline and aerobic training in patients with migraine.	- Weekly telephone calls to assess the progress of training. - One supervised training session. - Explanatory leaflet about the warm-up exercises.	18
Madsen, 2018 [60]	60 [68%], 32 ± Na	To examine the effectiveness of resistance training and postural exercise on tension-type headache frequency and duration.	- Weekly telephone calls to assess the progress of training. - Some supervised training sessions. - An exercise diary to monitor adherence and migraine intensity.	19
Mehta, 2021 [61]	61 [74%], 39 ± 8.24	To evaluate and compare the effectiveness of physical and yoga therapies in patients with migraine.	- Weekly telephone calls to assess the progress of training. - Some supervised training sessions. - An exercise diary to monitor adherence.	19

F: female; SD: standard deviation; and Na: not available.

3.2. Methodological Quality

For each study, the methodological quality was analysed through the modified version of the Downs and Black Checklist. All studies included were rated as "fair quality" [59–61]. These results must consider that some items on the checklist are difficult to use in sport and exercise field. For example, the use of a double-blind study design is difficult due to the presence of a program with physical activity.

3.3. Aerobic Training

Among the identified studies that used aerobic training, there is the article by Santiago and colleagues [59]. Researchers evaluated the benefits induced by the association between exercise and medication compared to medication alone in patients with migraine. The inclusion criteria for this study were a diagnosis of chronic migraine, normal cardiac and neurological examination, and being sedentary for at least 3 months. Based on these criteria, 60 patients were included and divided into two groups: a control group receiving pharmacological treatment only, and an experimental group combining pharmacological treatment with a TC training program. The control group was treated with amitriptyline (25 mg/day) for 12 weeks. The experimental group followed the same pharmacological treatment but integrated with an aerobic training program. The aerobic training program, performed via TC, consisted of free outdoor walking of 40 min with a weekly frequency of 3 times for 12 consecutive weeks. TC strategies included weekly phone calls to monitor progress and motivate participants, the flexibility for participants to choose when and where to perform the exercises, a spreadsheet with a detailed training plan to ensure the correct execution of the exercises, and a supervised training session with a movement expert. The following parameters were evaluated: frequency (days/month), intensity, and duration/day of migraine attacks (6 h, 12 h, 18 h, and 24 h), body mass index, Back Depression Inventory, and Beck Anxiety Inventory at baseline and the end of the third month. Both groups showed a decrease in the frequency, intensity, and duration of migraine episodes. However, the efficacy of amitriptyline increased when combined with the TC training program.

3.4. Resistance Training

Of the identified studies, Madsen and colleagues [60] used a TC approach to examine the effectiveness of a resistance training program and a postural training program on the frequency and duration of migraine. A total of 60 subjects were randomised into two groups: the control group and the experimental group. The control group was instructed on ergonomic and postural correction and performed postural exercises three times a day for 10 weeks. The experimental group performed a resistance training program, with three sessions per week for 10 weeks. The resistance training program involved the execution of specific shoulder exercises with progressive intensity: initially 70%, and later 80% of 1RM. All exercises were performed with elastic bands. TC approach was applied in both groups and the strategies included a free choice of when and where to perform the exercises, weekly calls to monitor exercise adherence and manage progress and motivate subjects to protocol adherence, and some supervised sessions to manage the correct execution of exercises. In addition, participants were given a migraine diary to record the frequency, duration, and intensity of headache episodes. Although no statistically significant changes were detected between groups, the experimental group reduced the frequency of headache episodes by 11% and the duration by 10%, while the control group showed a 24% reduction in frequency and 27% in duration 27% of headache attacks.

3.5. Physical Therapy

Mehta and colleagues [61] used a randomised controlled trial to evaluate and compare the effectiveness of physical therapy (stretching) and yoga therapies, applied with a TC approach, for the adjuvant therapy of standard pharmacologic treatment in patients with migraine. Subjects diagnosed with migraine, over 18 years old, and with at least five headache attacks per month were included in the study. A total of 61 patients were distributed in three groups: physical therapy, yoga therapy, and standard therapy. The physical therapy group practiced relaxation exercises, stretching of the neck muscles, and cardiorespiratory endurance training (30 min of free walking). The yoga therapy group performed several specific exercises, including the position of the butterfly (Bhadrasana), the position of the cobra (Bhunjagasana), and the touch of the feet standing (Padhastasana). The standard treatment group continued the usual medication treatment without any additional physical therapy. Participants performed the specific program for 12 weeks. All subjects received lifestyle advice including obtaining adequate rest, not skipping meals, avoiding bright lights, and using a headache diary to identify headache triggers. TC strategies, both physical therapy and yoga groups, included free choice of when and where to perform the exercises, constant weekly calls to monitor the progress, encouragement for participants, and motivation for them to perform the recommended intervention regularly. All groups showed statistically significant improvements in the frequency and severity of headaches. Additionally, pain assessments revealed improvements in all groups compared to baseline.

Table 3 summarises the different types of treatment and the training programs applied to the TC approach.

Table 3. Types of program in telecoaching.

Author, Years	Exercise	Intervention (n)	Program (time)	Training Program	Main Results
Santiago, 2014 [59]	AT	TCG (30) vs. CG (30)	12 weeks of training, 3 times/W	TCG: 40' free outdoor walk. CG: usual daily activities + drug treatment.	The drug was an effective treatment for chronic migraine, but its efficacy was increased when combined with AT.
Madsen, 2018 [60]	RT	TCG_1 (30) vs. TCG_2 (30)	10 weeks of training, 3 times/W	TCG_1: shoulder exercises with resistance from the elastic bands. TCG_2: ergonomic and posture correction + specific exercise for lumbar lordosis.	Both groups showed a reduction in the frequency and duration of migraine episodes.
Mehta, 2021 [61]	PT	TCG_1 (20) vs. TCG_2 (20) vs. CG (21)	12 weeks of training, 4 times/W	TCG_1: progressive muscle relaxation exercise, self-stretching of neck muscles, isometric exercise of neck muscles, and cardiorespiratory endurance training (30' free walking). TCG_2: Pranayama, and asana followed by Savasana. CG: usual daily activities.	Physical therapy and yoga, added to regular care, improved QoL and reduced the frequency of migraine.

TCG: telecoaching group; CG: control group; W: week; QoL: quality of life; AT: aerobic training; RT: resistance training; and PT: physical therapy.

4. Discussion

The primary aim of this scoping review was to investigate the use and feasibility of TC training programs in patients with migraine. The main outcomes assessed included the intensity, frequency, and duration of headache episodes, as well as pain perception and any potential adverse events. The present study showed very interesting results. First, this scoping review comprised more than 60% of women, a distribution that aligns with numerous epidemiological studies reporting a female to male ratio of 3:1 [62]. Second, the review demonstrated that in the analysed studies, an exercise conducted in TC significantly reduced the burden of headache attacks, leading to decreases in their intensity, frequency, and duration.

4.1. The Benefits of Physical Exercise in Migraine Management

The relationship between exercise and migraine is very complex [63]. Many studies show how physical exercise may represent a trigger for migraine attacks [18,64]. Nevertheless, for many authors, these negative aspects would depend on the excessive intensity of exercise [20] or performing an inadequate warm-up [65]. We can hypothesise that it may depend on the rise of serum calcitonin gene-related peptide (CGRP) levels occurring during exercise for its cardiovascular role in vasodilation [66,67] in a susceptible subject. In contrast, many studies highlight the positive effects of exercise in this population. Indeed, exercise would seem to significantly reduce the impact of migraine, improving the lifestyle and QoL [68,69]. Moreover, the absence of exercise, which increased during the COVID-19 pandemic and related social restrictions, has been shown to affect sleep quality in migraineurs [70]. The benefits of physical exercise would seem to depend on an increase in the plasma level of β-endorphins [71]; in fact, the β-endorphin level appears to be lower in migraineurs than in healthy subjects [72]. There is evidence that exercise increases the concentration of β-endorphins in healthy individuals [73,74]. Köseoglu and colleagues [75] showed a similar effect on migraine patients both after a single training session and after a prolonged training program. Further studies in the literature highlight additional benefits of exercise in this population, including increased cardiovascular and cerebrovascular capacity, as well as improvements in psychological states such as depression, stress, and anxiety [63,76]. Moreover, exercise has been shown to improve pain perception [77]. After exercise, patients show a reduction in pain-related fear and its perception [77]. In addition, migraine is a risk factor for excessive drug intake [78]. Overuse of medications in migraine patients causes increased disability, depression, anxiety, and fear, as well as increased pain and headache frequency (i.e., medication overuse headache) [79]. Consequently, exercise can be proposed as a useful tool to counteract the high use of drugs. Despite these positive aspects, as shown by Lemmens and colleagues [80], the drop-out rate to exercise is very high in migraineurs, due to the lack of time to perform supervised exercise training sessions/week [80].

4.2. Telecoaching: A Digital Approach to Migraine Management

Considering the spread and convenience of telemedicine, the new technological solutions in managing migraine [81], along with the need for structural changes in healthcare [82], TC could represent a valuable approach for this population. By providing personalised guidance and remote support, TC aligns with modern healthcare trends and has the potential to enhance adherence to physical activity programs. This approach could be particularly beneficial for migraine patients, offering accessible and flexible training options that remove common barriers to exercise. However, it is important to acknowledge the psychological variables and the strong association between anxiety, mood disorders, depression, and migraine [83]. Participants' attitudes toward TC may have played a crucial role in their performance in the included studies [82]. Positive attitudes toward this training modality can improve participant engagement, adherence, and overall satisfaction, while negative perceptions may reduce participation and limit the effectiveness of the intervention. This highlights the need to design user-friendly tools and methods that support acceptance of the condition and provide adaptive content and functionality [82]. However, attitudes toward telemedicine and eHealth are rarely reported or analysed as factors influencing participant performance in existing studies [84]. Future research should address this gap by incorporating these attitudes as a variable of interest, both in study design and analysis. To reduce stress, a major trigger of migraine attacks, Varkey and colleagues proposed the implementation of home training programs [85], incorporating TC training modality to enhance physical activity levels. Consistent with Varkey's study [85], the articles included in this review have shown several benefits. Indeed, in every study included in this review, the dropout rate in the TC group did not exceed 30%, with one study that showed a 0% dropout rate for the TC training program [61]. This demonstrates how TC is a sustainable and accepted training methodology in this population. This finding is significant for patients who intend to perform a training protocol and for physicians who intend to advise active participation in a physical activity program for migraine patients. The sustainability of TC and the relative benefits (i.e., training in the preferred place, during the leisure time, breaking down barriers such as costs and structures [37]) make TC one of the main solutions for physical activity intervention. The sustainability of TC in migraine is in line with the scientific literature for other neurological diseases. Burns and colleagues evaluated the effectiveness of a TC resistance training program for the weakness of the dorsiflexion of the foot in children with Charcot–Marie–Tooth polyneuropathy. The intervention program attenuated the progression of weakness in dorsiflexion without side effects and with a low abandonment rate (8%) [44]. Van der Kolk and colleagues evaluated the efficacy of aerobic exercise performed in TC to relieve motor symptoms in patients with mild-severity PD. The reduction in motor symptoms demonstrated in the intervention group showed how TC can be a useful additional tool to manage this disease. Ninety-four percent of the participants completed the study, demonstrating high tolerance to the TC training modality. In agreement with Varkey and colleagues, our study suggests the possible implementation of TC in patients with migraine; although, the few included studies reported in this scoping review do not allow us to evaluate in detail the relationship between TC and migraine in detail. Future studies should analyse and evaluate the efficacy of a fully executed TC training program, using uniform outcome measures for migraine as recommended by the International Headache Society [86], with a randomised controlled trial design based on the guidelines of the American College of Sports Medicine (3–5 days per week, 20–60 min, with an intensity equal to 55/65–90% of maximum heart rate).

4.3. Strength and Limitations

The following limitations were identified in this study: firstly, the few studies included and the heterogeneity of the physical activity programs used could alter the generalisation of results, not allowing the correct relationship between migraine and TC to be assessed. Secondly, the quality of the studies was not excellent, a condition that could depend on the researchers' lack of double-blinding (a condition that is difficult to apply with an exercise program to be performed). Additionally, the lack of homogeneity in the evaluation methods did not allow us to conduct a meta-analysis. Finally, the absence of a direct comparison between groups treated with and without TC represents a significant limitation of this review, as it does not allow us to assess in detail the true effects of TC. Thus, the observed benefits may not be exclusively attributed to TC.

Future studies should aim to design randomised controlled trials to clarify these effects and to evaluate the participant's attitudes towards the TC, especially considering the absence of psychological component evaluations in the included studies. Despite these limitations, this review has several strengths. It highlights that TC is potentially safe, effective, and risk-free for migraine patients. An additional strength is the dropout rate: no included study showed a dropout exceeding 30% and one study noted a 0% dropout rate. Finally, to our knowledge, this is the first review in the literature to examine the application of TC in migraine patients, as well as the first attempt to evaluate novel treatments for the management of this disease and the exacerbation of symptoms observed during the COVID-19 pandemic [87].

5. Conclusions

The results of this review, based on GRADE guidelines, show low evidence that exercise performed in TC is beneficial in patients with migraine. Further studies are needed to show the efficacy, benefits, and safety of this training modality, as well as to establish guidelines for administering a TC training program in this population. Future research should focus on high-quality randomised controlled trials to clarify and isolate the effects of TC on migraine outcomes. These studies should aim to standardise physical activity programs and standardised outcome measures to enable more comparisons. Additionally, it is essential to assess participants' attitudes toward TC in future studies, as this factor could significantly influence their performance and engagement. Addressing these gaps will help to clarify the role of TC as a treatment modality for migraine and establish evidence-based guidelines for its use.

Author Contributions: Conceptualization, G.B. and I.L.; methodology, I.L.; software, I.L. and V.D.S.; validation, V.D.S.; formal analysis, I.L. and V.D.S.; investigation, I.L. and V.D.S.; resources, A.T.; data curation, I.L.; writing—original draft preparation, I.L. and V.D.S.; writing—review and editing, G.B., V.G., R.M., P.A., M.R. and A.T.; visualization, I.L.; supervision, G.B. and F.B.; project administration, G.B. All authors have read and agreed to the published version of the manuscript.

Funding: This research received no external funding.

Conflicts of Interest: The authors declare no conflict of interest.

References

1. Stovner, L.J.; Andree, C. Prevalence of headache in Europe: A review for the Eurolight project. *J. Headache Pain* **2010**, *11*, 289–299. [CrossRef] [PubMed]
2. Steiner, T.J.; Stovner, L.J.; Vos, T.; Jensen, R.; Katsarava, Z. Migraine is first cause of disability in under 50s: Will health politicians now take notice? *J. Headache Pain* **2018**, *19*, 17. [CrossRef] [PubMed]
3. Headache Classification Committee of the International Headache Society (IHS). The International Classification of Headache Disorders, 3rd edition. *Cephalalgia* **2018**, *38*, 1–211. [CrossRef] [PubMed]
4. Leonardi, M.; Raggi, A.; Ajovalasit, D.; Bussone, G.; D'Amico, D. Functioning and disability in migraine. *Disabil. Rehabil.* **2010**, *32* (Suppl. S1), S23–S32. [CrossRef]
5. Linde, M.; Gustavsson, A.; Stovner, L.J.; Steiner, T.J.; Barré, J.; Katsarava, Z.; Lainez, J.M.; Lampl, C.; Lantéri-Minet, M.; Rastenyte, D.; et al. The cost of headache disorders in Europe: The Eurolight project. *Eur. J. Neurol.* **2012**, *19*, 703–711. [CrossRef]
6. Evers, S.; Afra, J.; Frese, A.; Goadsby, P.J.; Linde, M.; May, A.; Sándor, P.S. EFNS guideline on the drug treatment of migraine—Revised report of an EFNS task force. *Eur. J. Neurol.* **2009**, *16*, 968–981. [CrossRef]
7. Brighina, F.; Palermo, A.; Daniele, O.; Aloisio, A.; Fierro, B. High-frequency transcranial magnetic stimulation on motor cortex of patients affected by migraine with aura: A way to restore normal cortical excitability? *Cephalalgia* **2010**, *30*, 46–52. [CrossRef]
8. Viganò, A.; Toscano, M.; Puledda, F.; Di Piero, V. Treating Chronic Migraine with Neuromodulation: The Role of Neurophysiological Abnormalities and Maladaptive Plasticity. *Front. Pharmacol.* **2019**, *10*, 32. [CrossRef]
9. Cosentino, G.; Fierro, B.; Vigneri, S.; Talamanca, S.; Paladino, P.; Baschi, R.; Indovino, S.; Maccora, S.; Valentino, F.; Fileccia, E.; et al. Cyclical changes of cortical excitability and metaplasticity in migraine: Evidence from a repetitive transcranial magnetic stimulation study. *Pain* **2014**, *155*, 1070–1078. [CrossRef]
10. Di Stefano, V.; Rispoli, M.G.; Pellegrino, N.; Graziosi, A.; Rotondo, E.; Napoli, C.; Pietrobon, D.; Brighina, F.; Parisi, P. Diagnostic and therapeutic aspects of hemiplegic migraine. *J. Neurol. Neurosurg. Psychiatry* **2020**, *91*, 764–771. [CrossRef]
11. Brighina, F.; Cosentino, G.; Vigneri, S.; Talamanca, S.; Palermo, A.; Giglia, G.; Fierro, B. Abnormal facilitatory mechanisms in motor cortex of migraine with aura. *Eur. J. Pain* **2011**, *15*, 928–935. [CrossRef] [PubMed]
12. Eigenbrodt, A.K.; Ashina, H.; Khan, S.; Diener, H.C.; Mitsikostas, D.D.; Sinclair, A.J.; Pozo-Rosich, P.; Martelletti, P.; Ducros, A.; Lantéri-Minet, M.; et al. Diagnosis and management of migraine in ten steps. *Nat. Rev. Neurol.* **2021**, *17*, 501–514. [CrossRef] [PubMed]
13. Marmura, M.J.; Silberstein, S.D.; Schwedt, T.J. The acute treatment of migraine in adults: The american headache society evidence assessment of migraine pharmacotherapies. *Headache* **2015**, *55*, 3–20. [CrossRef] [PubMed]
14. Kowacs, P.A.; Piovesan, E.J.; Tepper, S.J. Rejection and acceptance of possible side effects of migraine prophylactic drugs. *Headache* **2009**, *49*, 1022–1027. [CrossRef]
15. Koseoglu, E.; Yetkin, M.F.; Ugur, F.; Bilgen, M. The role of exercise in migraine treatment. *J. Sports Med. Phys. Fitness* **2015**, *55*, 1029–1036.
16. Chaibi, A.; Tuchin, P.J.; Russell, M.B. Manual therapies for migraine: A systematic review. *J. Headache Pain* **2011**, *12*, 127–133. [CrossRef]
17. Probyn, K.; Bowers, H.; Mistry, D.; Caldwell, F.; Underwood, M.; Patel, S.; Sandhu, H.K.; Matharu, M.; Pincus, T. Non-pharmacological self-management for people living with migraine or tension-type headache: A systematic review including analysis of intervention components. *BMJ Open* **2017**, *7*, e016670. [CrossRef]
18. Amin, F.M.; Aristeidou, S.; Baraldi, C.; Czapinska-Ciepiela, E.K.; Ariadni, D.D.; Di Lenola, D.; Fenech, C.; Kampouris, K.; Karagiorgis, G.; Braschinsky, M.; et al. The association between migraine and physical exercise. *J. Headache Pain* **2018**, *19*, 83. [CrossRef]
19. Pilati, L.; Battaglia, G.; Di Stefano, V.; Di Marco, S.; Torrente, A.; Raieli, V.; Firenze, A.; Salemi, G.; Brighina, F. Migraine and Sport in a Physically Active Population of Students: Results of a Cross-Sectional Study. *Headache* **2020**, *60*, 2330–2339. [CrossRef]
20. Hougaard, A.; Amin, F.M.; Hauge, A.W.; Ashina, M.; Olesen, J. Provocation of migraine with aura using natural trigger factors. *Neurology* **2013**, *80*, 428–431. [CrossRef]
21. Hauge, A.W.; Kirchmann, M.; Olesen, J. Trigger factors in migraine with aura. *Cephalalgia* **2010**, *30*, 346–353. [CrossRef] [PubMed]

22. Varkey, E.; Cider, A.; Carlsson, J.; Linde, M. Exercise as migraine prophylaxis: A randomized study using relaxation and topiramate as controls. *Cephalalgia* **2011**, *31*, 1428–1434. [CrossRef] [PubMed]
23. Busch, V.; Gaul, C. Exercise in migraine therapy--is there any evidence for efficacy? A critical review. *Headache* **2008**, *48*, 890–899. [CrossRef] [PubMed]
24. Borisovskaya, A.; Chmelik, E.; Karnik, A. Exercise and Chronic Pain. *Adv. Exp. Med. Biol.* **2020**, *1228*, 233–253. [CrossRef]
25. Fernández-Rodríguez, R.; Álvarez-Bueno, C.; Cavero-Redondo, I.; Torres-Costoso, A.; Pozuelo-Carrascosa, D.P.; Reina-Gutiérrez, S.; Pascual-Morena, C.; Martínez-Vizcaíno, V. Best Exercise Options for Reducing Pain and Disability in Adults With Chronic Low Back Pain: Pilates, Strength, Core-Based, and Mind-Body. A Network Meta-analysis. *J. Orthop. Sports Phys. Ther.* **2022**, *52*, 505–521. [CrossRef]
26. Varkey, E.; Hagen, K.; Zwart, J.A.; Linde, M. Physical activity and headache: Results from the Nord-Trøndelag Health Study (HUNT). *Cephalalgia* **2008**, *28*, 1292–1297. [CrossRef]
27. Leale, I.; Giustino, V.; Trapani, P.; Alonge, P.; Rini, N.; Cutrò, I.; Leone, O.; Torrente, A.; Lupica, A.; Palma, A.; et al. Physical Activity in Patients with Neuromuscular Disease Three Years after COVID-19, a Longitudinal Survey: The After-Effects of the Quarantine and the Benefits of a Return to a Healthier Life-Style. *J. Clin. Med.* **2024**, *13*, 265. [CrossRef]
28. Di Stefano, V.; Battaglia, G.; Giustino, V.; Gagliardo, A.; D'Aleo, M.; Giannini, O.; Palma, A.; Brighina, F. Significant reduction of physical activity in patients with neuromuscular disease during COVID-19 pandemic: The long-term consequences of quarantine. *J. Neurol.* **2021**, *268*, 20–26. [CrossRef]
29. Narin, S.O.; Pinar, L.; Erbas, D.; Oztürk, V.; Idiman, F. The effects of exercise and exercise-related changes in blood nitric oxide level on migraine headache. *Clin. Rehabil.* **2003**, *17*, 624–630. [CrossRef]
30. Lockett, D.M.; Campbell, J.F. The effects of aerobic exercise on migraine. *Headache* **1992**, *32*, 50–54. [CrossRef]
31. Reina-Varona, Á.; Madroñero-Miguel, B.; Fierro-Marrero, J.; Paris-Alemany, A.; La Touche, R. Efficacy of various exercise interventions for migraine treatment: A systematic review and network meta-analysis. *Headache J. Head Face Pain* **2024**, *64*, 873–900. [CrossRef] [PubMed]
32. Woldeamanuel, Y.W.; Oliveira, A.B.D. What is the efficacy of aerobic exercise versus strength training in the treatment of migraine? A systematic review and network meta-analysis of clinical trials. *J. Headache Pain* **2022**, *23*, 134. [CrossRef] [PubMed]
33. Zhao, H.; Cheng, R.; Song, G.; Teng, J.; Shen, S.; Fu, X.; Yan, Y.; Liu, C. The Effect of Resistance Training on the Rehabilitation of Elderly Patients with Sarcopenia: A Meta-Analysis. *Int. J. Environ. Res. Public Health* **2022**, *19*, 15491. [CrossRef] [PubMed]
34. Caverni, C.N.; da Costa, A.T.; Simioni, C.G.; Fukue, R.R.; Tengan, C.H.; Villa, T.R. Evaluation of body composition in patients with migraine on prophylactic treatment with topiramate. *Heliyon* **2021**, *7*, e06765. [CrossRef]
35. Ha, W.S.; Kim, J.; Hwang, H.W.; Lee, S.H.; Kim, J.I.; Hong, J.Y.; Park, S.H.; Han, K.D.; Baek, M.S. The association between migraine and Parkinson's disease: A nationwide cohort study. *Epidemiol. Health* **2024**, *46*, e2024010. [CrossRef]
36. Kim, J.; Ha, W.S.; Park, S.H.; Han, K.; Baek, M.S. Association between migraine and Alzheimer's disease: A nationwide cohort study. *Front. Aging Neurosci.* **2023**, *15*, 1196185. [CrossRef]
37. University, C.S. Telecoaching Emerges as Tool in Nutrition and Medicine. Available online: https://source.colostate.edu/telecoaching-emerges-as-tool-in-nutrition-and-medicine/ (accessed on 19 October 2024).
38. Leale, I.; Figlioli, F.; Giustino, V.; Brusa, J.; Barcellona, M.; Nocera, V.; Canzone, A.; Patti, A.; Messina, G.; Barbagallo, M.; et al. Telecoaching as a new training method for elderly people: A systematic review. *Aging Clin. Exp. Res.* **2024**, *36*, 18. [CrossRef]
39. Leale, I.; Giustino, V.; Brusa, J.; Barcellona, M.; Barbagallo, M.; Palma, A.; Messina, G.; Dominguez, L.J.; Battaglia, G. Effectiveness of a Sustainable Training Program Combining Supervised Outdoor Exercise with Telecoaching on Physical Performance in Elderly People. *Sustainability* **2024**, *16*, 3254. [CrossRef]
40. Cameron-Tucker, H.L.; Wood-Baker, R.; Joseph, L.; Walters, J.A.; Schüz, N.; Walters, E.H. A randomized controlled trial of telephone-mentoring with home-based walking preceding rehabilitation in COPD. *Int. J. Chronic Obstr. Pulm. Dis.* **2016**, *11*, 1991–2000. [CrossRef]
41. Hume, E.; Muse, H.; Wallace, K.; Wilkinson, M.; Heslop Marshall, K.; Nair, A.; Clark, S.; Vogiatzis, I. Feasibility and acceptability of a physical activity behavioural modification tele-coaching intervention in lung transplant recipients. *Chronic Respir. Dis.* **2022**, *19*, 14799731221116588. [CrossRef]
42. De Vasconcelos, H.C.A.; Lira Neto, J.C.G.; De Araújo, M.F.M.; Carvalho, G.C.N.; De Souza Teixeira, C.R.; De Freitas, R.W.J.F.; Damasceno, M.M.C. Telecoaching programme for type 2 diabetes control: A randomised clinical trial. *Br. J. Nurs.* **2018**, *27*, 1115–1120. [CrossRef] [PubMed]
43. Snoek, J.A.; Meindersma, E.P.; Prins, L.F.; van't Hof, A.W.J.; de Boer, M.J.; Hopman, M.T.; Eijsvogels, T.M.H.; de Kluiver, E.P. The sustained effects of extending cardiac rehabilitation with a six-month telemonitoring and telecoaching programme on fitness, quality of life, cardiovascular risk factors and care utilisation in CAD patients: The TeleCaRe study. *J. Telemed. Telecare* **2021**, *27*, 473–483. [CrossRef] [PubMed]

44. Burns, J.; Sman, A.D.; Cornett, K.M.D.; Wojciechowski, E.; Walker, T.; Menezes, M.P.; Mandarakas, M.R.; Rose, K.J.; Bray, P.; Sampaio, H.; et al. Safety and efficacy of progressive resistance exercise for Charcot-Marie-Tooth disease in children: A randomised, double-blind, sham-controlled trial. *Lancet Child Adolesc. Health* **2017**, *1*, 106–113. [CrossRef] [PubMed]
45. Leale, I.; Di Stefano, V.; Costanza, C.; Brighina, F.; Roccella, M.; Palma, A.; Battaglia, G. Telecoaching: A potential new training model for Charcot-Marie-Tooth patients: A systematic review. *Front. Neurol.* **2024**, *15*, 1359091. [CrossRef]
46. Irby, M.B.; Bond, D.S.; Lipton, R.B.; Nicklas, B.; Houle, T.T.; Penzien, D.B. Aerobic Exercise for Reducing Migraine Burden: Mechanisms, Markers, and Models of Change Processes. *Headache* **2016**, *56*, 357–369. [CrossRef]
47. Clausen, T.C.; Greve, N.K.; Müller, K.I.; Kristoffersen, E.S.; Schytz, H.W. Telemedicine in headache care: A systematic review. *Cephalalgia* **2022**, *42*, 1397–1408. [CrossRef]
48. Noutsios, C.D.; Boisvert-Plante, V.; Perez, J.; Hudon, J.; Ingelmo, P. Telemedicine Applications for the Evaluation of Patients with Non-Acute Headache: A Narrative Review. *J. Pain Res.* **2021**, *14*, 1533–1542. [CrossRef]
49. Giustino, V.; Leale, I.; Cicero, L.; Petrigna, L.; Lo Nigro, M.; Fontana, V.; Mignosi, E.; Cataldo, P.; Macaluso, A.; Gómez-López, M.; et al. Acute effects of a dog sport on fitness parameters in young adults: A randomised controlled crossover study. *Hum. Mov.* **2024**, *25*, 138–146. [CrossRef]
50. Kristoffersen, E.S.; Sandset, E.C.; Winsvold, B.S.; Faiz, K.W.; Storstein, A.M. Experiences of telemedicine in neurological out-patient clinics during the COVID-19 pandemic. *Ann. Clin. Transl. Neurol.* **2021**, *8*, 440–447. [CrossRef]
51. Andruskevicius, S.; Petrosian, D.; Dapkute, A.; Jokubaitis, M.; Ryliskiene, K. Evolving migraine management: Lithuania's telemedicine experience. *Front. Neurol.* **2024**, *15*, 1388100. [CrossRef]
52. Chiang, C.C.; Halker Singh, R.; Lalvani, N.; Shubin Stein, K.; Henscheid Lorenz, D.; Lay, C.; Dodick, D.W.; Newman, L.C. Patient experience of telemedicine for headache care during the COVID-19 pandemic: An American Migraine Foundation survey study. *Headache* **2021**, *61*, 734–739. [CrossRef] [PubMed]
53. Müller, K.I.; Alstadhaug, K.B.; Bekkelund, S.I. Acceptability, Feasibility, and Cost of Telemedicine for Nonacute Headaches: A Randomized Study Comparing Video and Traditional Consultations. *J. Med. Internet Res.* **2016**, *18*, e140. [CrossRef] [PubMed]
54. Shamseer, L.; Moher, D.; Clarke, M.; Ghersi, D.; Liberati, A.; Petticrew, M.; Shekelle, P.; Stewart, L.A. Preferred reporting items for systematic review and meta-analysis protocols (PRISMA-P) 2015: Elaboration and explanation. *BMJ* **2015**, *350*, g7647. [CrossRef] [PubMed]
55. Downs, S.H.; Black, N. The feasibility of creating a checklist for the assessment of the methodological quality both of randomised and non-randomised studies of health care interventions. *J. Epidemiol. Community Health* **1998**, *52*, 377–384. [CrossRef] [PubMed]
56. Chuter, V.; Spink, M.; Searle, A.; Ho, A. The effectiveness of shoe insoles for the prevention and treatment of low back pain: A systematic review and meta-analysis of randomised controlled trials. *BMC Musculoskelet. Disord.* **2014**, *15*, 140. [CrossRef]
57. Pas, H.I.; Reurink, G.; Tol, J.L.; Weir, A.; Winters, M.; Moen, M.H. Efficacy of rehabilitation (lengthening) exercises, platelet-rich plasma injections, and other conservative interventions in acute hamstring injuries: An updated systematic review and meta-analysis. *Br. J. Sports Med.* **2015**, *49*, 1197–1205. [CrossRef]
58. Hooper, P.; Jutai, J.W.; Strong, G.; Russell-Minda, E. Age-related macular degeneration and low-vision rehabilitation: A systematic review. *Can. J. Ophthalmol.* **2008**, *43*, 180–187. [CrossRef]
59. Santiago, M.D.; Carvalho Dde, S.; Gabbai, A.A.; Pinto, M.M.; Moutran, A.R.; Villa, T.R. Amitriptyline and aerobic exercise or amitriptyline alone in the treatment of chronic migraine: A randomized comparative study. *Arq. Neuro-Psiquiatr.* **2014**, *72*, 851–855. [CrossRef]
60. Madsen, B.K.; Søgaard, K.; Andersen, L.L.; Tornøe, B.; Jensen, R.H. Efficacy of strength training on tension-type headache: A randomised controlled study. *Cephalalgia* **2018**, *38*, 1071–1080. [CrossRef]
61. Mehta, J.N.; Parikh, S.; Desai, S.D.; Solanki, R.C.; Pathak, A.G. Study of Additive Effect of Yoga and Physical Therapies to Standard Pharmacologic Treatment in Migraine. *J. Neurosci. Rural. Pract.* **2021**, *12*, 60–66. [CrossRef]
62. Moens, G.; Johannik, K.; Verbeek, C.; Bulterys, S. The prevalence and characteristics of migraine among the Belgian working population. *Acta Neurol. Belg.* **2007**, *107*, 84–90. [PubMed]
63. Darling, M. Exercise and migraine. A critical review. *J. Sports Med. Phys. Fit.* **1991**, *31*, 294–302.
64. Annalisa, G.; Davide, B.; Marco, A. Sport and migraine-a dynamic relationship. *Neurol. Sci.* **2022**, *43*, 5749–5751. [CrossRef] [PubMed]
65. Lambert, R.W., Jr.; Burnet, D.L. Prevention of exercise induced migraine by quantitative warm-up. *Headache* **1985**, *25*, 317–319. [CrossRef]
66. Lind, H.; Brudin, L.; Lindholm, L.; Edvinsson, L. Different levels of sensory neuropeptides (calcitonin gene-related peptide and substance P) during and after exercise in man. *Clin. Physiol.* **1996**, *16*, 73–82. [CrossRef]
67. Onuoha, G.N.; Nicholls, D.P.; Patterson, A.; Beringer, T. Neuropeptide secretion in exercise. *Neuropeptides* **1998**, *32*, 319–325. [CrossRef]
68. Hagen, K.; Wisløff, U.; Ellingsen, Ø.; Stovner, L.J.; Linde, M. Headache and peak oxygen uptake: The HUNT3 study. *Cephalalgia* **2015**, *36*, 437–444. [CrossRef]

69. La Touche, R.; Fernández Pérez, J.J.; Proy Acosta, A.; González Campodónico, L.; Martínez García, S.; Adraos Juárez, D.; Serrano García, B.; Angulo-Díaz-Parreño, S.; Cuenca-Martínez, F.; Suso-Martí, L.; et al. Is aerobic exercise helpful in patients with migraine? A systematic review and meta-analysis. *Scand. J. Med. Sci. Sports* **2020**, *30*, 965–982. [CrossRef]
70. Di Stefano, V.; Ornello, R.; Gagliardo, A.; Torrente, A.; Illuminato, E.; Caponnetto, V.; Frattale, I.; Golini, R.; Di Felice, C.; Graziano, F.; et al. Social Distancing in Chronic Migraine during the COVID-19 Outbreak: Results from a Multicenter Observational Study. *Nutrients* **2021**, *13*, 1361. [CrossRef]
71. Pertovaara, A.; Huopaniemi, T.; Virtanen, A.; Johansson, G. The influence of exercise on dental pain thresholds and the release of stress hormones. *Physiol. Behav.* **1984**, *33*, 923–926. [CrossRef]
72. Misra, U.K.; Kalita, J.; Tripathi, G.M.; Bhoi, S.K. Is β endorphin related to migraine headache and its relief? *Cephalalgia* **2013**, *33*, 316–322. [CrossRef] [PubMed]
73. Pierce, E.F.; Eastman, N.W.; Tripathi, H.L.; Olson, K.G.; Dewey, W.L. Beta-endorphin response to endurance exercise: Relationship to exercise dependence. *Percept. Mot. Ski.* **1993**, *77*, 767–770. [CrossRef] [PubMed]
74. Grossman, A.; Sutton, J.R. Endorphins: What are they? How are they measured? What is their role in exercise? *Med. Sci. Sports Exerc.* **1985**, *17*, 74–81. [CrossRef]
75. Köseoglu, E.; Akboyraz, A.; Soyuer, A.; Ersoy, A. Aerobic Exercise and Plasma Beta Endorphin Levels in Patients with Migrainous Headache Without Aura. *Cephalalgia* **2003**, *23*, 972–976. [CrossRef]
76. Ledwidge, B. Run for your mind: Aerobic exercise as a means of alleviating anxiety and depression. *Can. J. Behav. Sci./Rev. Can. Des Sci. Comport.* **1980**, *12*, 126–140. [CrossRef]
77. Smith, B.E.; Hendrick, P.; Bateman, M.; Holden, S.; Littlewood, C.; Smith, T.O.; Logan, P. Musculoskeletal pain and exercise—Challenging existing paradigms and introducing new. *Br. J. Sports Med.* **2019**, *53*, 907. [CrossRef]
78. Hagen, K.; Linde, M.; Steiner, T.J.; Stovner, L.J.; Zwart, J.A. Risk factors for medication-overuse headache: An 11-year follow-up study. The Nord-Trøndelag Health Studies. *Pain* **2012**, *153*, 56–61. [CrossRef]
79. Peck, K.R.; Roland, M.M.; Smitherman, T.A. Factors Associated With Medication-Overuse Headache in Patients Seeking Treatment for Primary Headache. *Headache J. Head Face Pain* **2018**, *58*, 648–660. [CrossRef]
80. Lemmens, J.; De Pauw, J.; Van Soom, T.; Michiels, S.; Versijpt, J.; Van Breda, E.; Castien, R.; De Hertogh, W. The effect of aerobic exercise on the number of migraine days, duration and pain intensity in migraine: A systematic literature review and meta-analysis. *J. Headache Pain* **2019**, *20*, 16. [CrossRef]
81. Liu, Q.; Liu, F.; Yu, X.; Zang, J.; Tan, G. Telemedicine efficacy and satisfaction of patients and headache specialists in migraine management. *Front. Mol. Neurosci.* **2023**, *16*, 1093287. [CrossRef]
82. Brzeskot Ganning, E. Designing Migraine Applications: A Qualitative Interview Study on Migraine Patients' Motivation of using Mhealth Applications. Master's Thesis, Linköping University, Linköping, Sweden, 2023.
83. Peres, M.F.P.; Mercante, J.P.P.; Tobo, P.R.; Kamei, H.; Bigal, M.E. Anxiety and depression symptoms and migraine: A symptom-based approach research. *J. Headache Pain* **2017**, *18*, 37. [CrossRef] [PubMed]
84. Giannouli, V.; Giannoulis, K. Better Understand to Better Predict Subjective Well-Being Among Older Greeks in COVID-19 Era: Depression, Anxiety, Attitudes Towards eHealth, Religiousness, Spiritual Experience, and Cognition. *Adv. Exp. Med. Biol.* **2023**, *1425*, 359–364. [CrossRef] [PubMed]
85. Varkey, E.; Cider, Å.; Carlsson, J.; Linde, M. A study to evaluate the feasibility of an aerobic exercise program in patients with migraine. *Headache* **2009**, *49*, 563–570. [CrossRef]
86. Tassorelli, C.; Diener, H.C.; Dodick, D.W.; Silberstein, S.D.; Lipton, R.B.; Ashina, M.; Becker, W.J.; Ferrari, M.D.; Goadsby, P.J.; Pozo-Rosich, P.; et al. Guidelines of the International Headache Society for controlled trials of preventive treatment of chronic migraine in adults. *Cephalalgia* **2018**, *38*, 815–832. [CrossRef]
87. Torrente, A.; Di Stefano, V. The Impact of COVID-19 on Migraine: The Patients' Perspective. *Life* **2024**, *14*, 1420. [CrossRef]

Disclaimer/Publisher's Note: The statements, opinions and data contained in all publications are solely those of the individual author(s) and contributor(s) and not of MDPI and/or the editor(s). MDPI and/or the editor(s) disclaim responsibility for any injury to people or property resulting from any ideas, methods, instructions or products referred to in the content.

MDPI AG
Grosspeteranlage 5
4052 Basel
Switzerland
Tel.: +41 61 683 77 34

Journal of Clinical Medicine Editorial Office
E-mail: jcm@mdpi.com
www.mdpi.com/journal/jcm

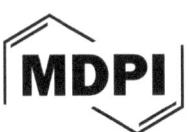

Disclaimer/Publisher's Note: The title and front matter of this reprint are at the discretion of the Guest Editors. The publisher is not responsible for their content or any associated concerns. The statements, opinions and data contained in all individual articles are solely those of the individual Editors and contributors and not of MDPI. MDPI disclaims responsibility for any injury to people or property resulting from any ideas, methods, instructions or products referred to in the content.

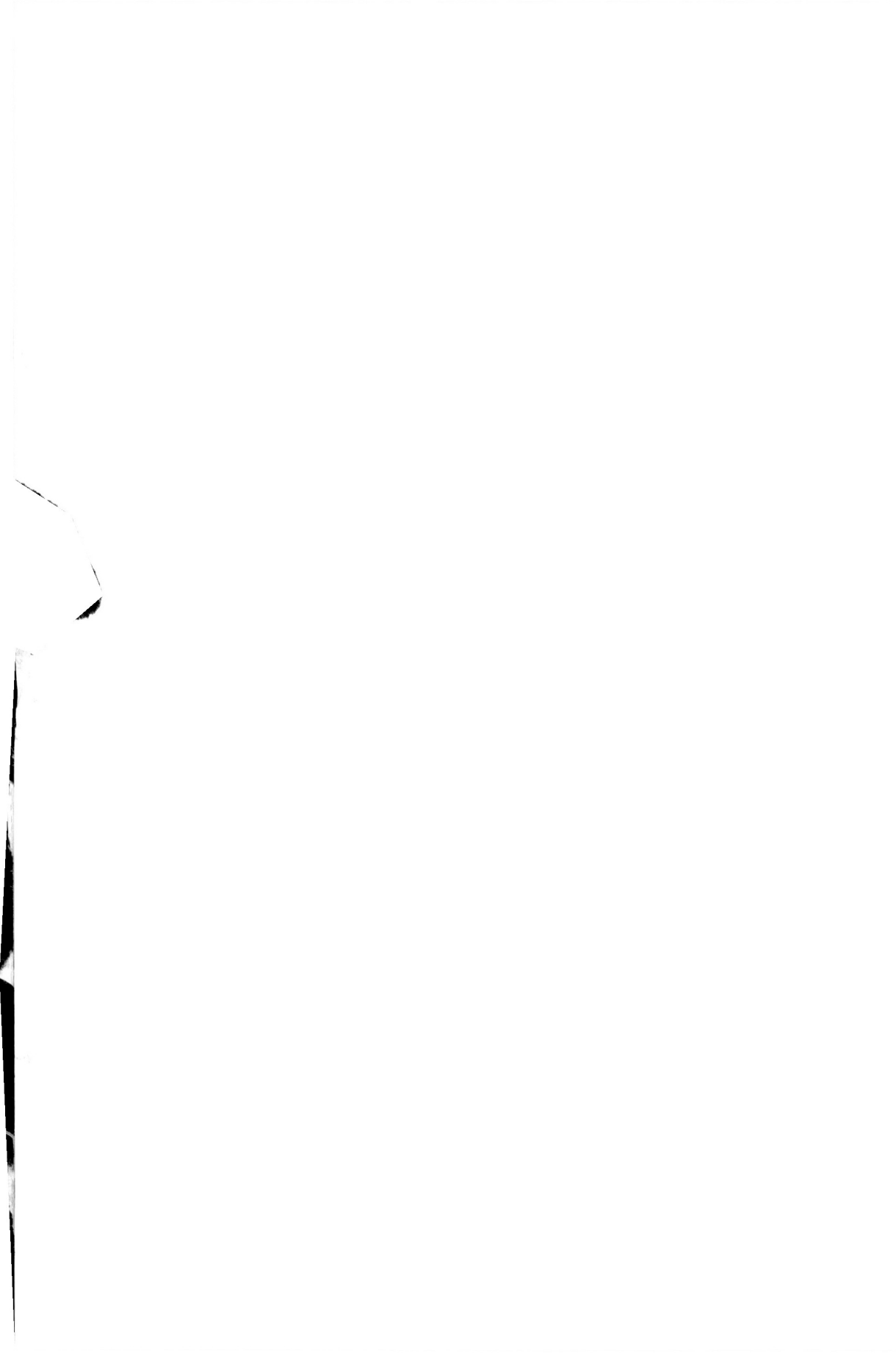

www.ingramcontent.com/pod-product-compliance
Lightning Source LLC
LaVergne TN
LVHW070002100526
838202LV00019B/2611